# Endodontics: Clinical and Scientific Updates

*Editor*

MO K. KANG

# DENTAL CLINICS OF NORTH AMERICA

www.dental.theclinics.com

January 2017 • Volume 61 • Number 1

**ELSEVIER**

1600 John F. Kennedy Boulevard • Suite 1800 • Philadelphia, Pennsylvania, 19103-2899

http://www.dental.theclinics.com

**DENTAL CLINICS OF NORTH AMERICA Volume 61, Number 1**
**January 2017 ISSN 0011-8532, ISBN: 978-0-323-48258-5**

Editor: John Vassallo; j.vassallo@elsevier.com
Developmental Editor: Kristen Helm

*Dental Clinics of North America* (ISSN 0011-8532) is published quarterly by Elsevier Inc., 360 Park Avenue South, New York, NY 10010-1710. Months of issue are January, April, July, and October. Business and Editorial Offices: 1600 John F. Kennedy Boulevard, Suite 1800, Philadelphia, PA 19103-2899. Periodicals postage paid at New York, NY and additional mailing offices. Subscription prices are $288.00 per year (domestic individuals), $569.00 per year (domestic institutions), $100.00 per year (domestic students/residents), $350.00 per year (Canadian individuals), $737.00 per year (Canadian institutions), $422.00 per year (international individuals), $737.00 per year (international institutions), and $200.00 per year (international and Canadian students/residents). International air speed delivery is included in all *Clinics* subscription prices. All prices are subject to change without notice. **POSTMASTER:** Send address changes to *Dental Clinics of North America*, Elsevier Health Sciences Division, Subscription Customer Service, 3251 Riverport Lane, Maryland Heights, MO 63043. **Customer Service (orders, claims, online, change of address): Elsevier Health Sciences Division, Subscription Customer Service, 3251 Riverport Lane, Maryland Heights, MO 63043. Tel: 1-800-654-2452 (U.S. and Canada). Fax: 314-447-8029. E-mail: journalscustomerservice-usa@elsevier.com (for print support); journalsonlinesupport-usa@elsevier.com (for online support).**

*Reprints.* For copies of 100 or more, of articles in this publication, please contact the Commercial Reprints Department, Elsevier Inc., 360 Park Avenue South, New York, NY 10010-1710. Tel.: 212-633-3874; Fax: 212-633-3820; E-mail: reprints@elsevier.com.

*The Dental Clinics of North America* is covered in *MEDLINE/PubMed (Index Medicus), Current Contents/Clinical Medicine, ISI/BIOMED* and *Clinahl*.

Printed in the United States of America.

# Contributors

## EDITOR

**MO K. KANG, DDS, PhD**
Diplomate, American Board of Endodontics; The Shapiro Family Laboratory of Viral Oncology and Aging Research, Professor and Chairman, Jack Weichman Endowed Chair, Section of Endodontics, Division of Constitutive and Regenerative Sciences, UCLA School of Dentistry, Los Angeles, California

## AUTHORS

**ABDULLAH ALSHAIKH, DDS**
The Shapiro Family Laboratory of Viral Oncology and Aging Research, Section of Endodontics, UCLA School of Dentistry, Los Angeles, California

**CHIDER CHEN, PhD**
Department of Anatomy and Cell Biology, School of Dental Medicine, University of Pennsylvania, Philadelphia, Pennsylvania

**BIN CHENG, PhD**
Associate Professor at Columbia University Medical Center, Department of Biostatistics, Columbia University Mailman School of Public Health, New York, New York

**NADIA CHUGAL, DDS, MS, MPH**
Diplomate, American Board of Endodontics; Clinical Professor; Program Director; Postdoctoral Endodontics, Section of Endodontics, UCLA School of Dentistry, Los Angeles, California

**MARIA GUIOMAR DE AZEVEDO BAHIA, DDS, MS, PhD**
Department of Restorative Dentistry, Faculty of Dentistry, Universidade Federal de Minas Gerais, Belo Horizonte, Minas Gerais, Brazil

**ANIBAL DIOGENES, DDS, MS, PhD**
Associate Professor, Department of Endodontics, University of Texas Health Science Center at San Antonio, San Antonio, Texas

**SPYROS FLORATOS, DMD**
Adjunct Assistant Professor, Department of Endodontics, University of Pennsylvania School of Dental Medicine, Philadelphia, Pennsylvania

**ASHRAF F. FOUAD, DDS, MS**
Freedland Distinguished Professor and Chair, Department of Endodontics, School of Dentistry, University of North Carolina, Chapel Hill, North Carolina

**QIMEI GONG, DDS, PhD**
Division of Endodontics, Center for Craniofacial Regeneration, Columbia University Medical Center, Columbia University, New York, New York; Department of Operative Dentistry and Endodontics, Guanghua School of Stomatology, Hospital of Stomatology, Guangdong Province Key Laboratory of Stomatology, Sun Yat-sen University, Guangzhou, Guangdong, China

**MARC HAYASHI, DMD**
Section of Restorative Dentistry, UCLA School of Dentistry, Los Angeles, California

**LING HE, DDS**
Division of Endodontics, Center for Craniofacial Regeneration, Columbia University Medical Center, Columbia University, New York, New York; Department of Operative Dentistry and Endodontics, Guanghua School of Stomatology, Hospital of Stomatology, Guangdong Province Key Laboratory of Stomatology, Sun Yat-sen University, Guangzhou, Guangdong, China

**BILL KAHLER, DClinDent, PhD**
School of Dentistry, The University of Queensland Oral Health Centre, Herston, Queensland, Australia

**MO K. KANG, DDS, PhD**
Diplomate, American Board of Endodontics; The Shapiro Family Laboratory of Viral Oncology and Aging Research, Professor and Chairman, Jack Weichman Endowed Chair, Section of Endodontics, Division of Constitutive and Regenerative Sciences, UCLA School of Dentistry, Los Angeles, California

**EUISEONG KIM, DDS, PhD**
Microscope Center, Department of Conservative Dentistry, Oral Science Research Center, Yonsei University College of Dentistry, Seoul, Korea

**REUBEN H. KIM, DDS, PhD**
The Shapiro Family Laboratory of Viral Oncology and Aging Research; Section of Restorative Dentistry, UCLA School of Dentistry, Los Angeles, California

**SAHNG G. KIM, DDS, MS**
Associate Professor of Dental Medicine at CUMC; Associate Professor, Division of Endodontics, Center for Craniofacial Regeneration, Columbia University Medical Center, College of Dental Medicine, Columbia University, New York, New York

**SOL KIM, PhD**
The Shapiro Family Laboratory of Viral Oncology and Aging Research; Section of Restorative Dentistry, UCLA School of Dentistry, Los Angeles, California

**SYNGCUK KIM, DDS, PhD, MD(Hon)**
Louis I Grossman Professor, Department of Endodontics, University of Pennsylvania School of Dental Medicine, Philadelphia, Pennsylvania

**JAMES LIM, DDS**
Section of Restorative Dentistry, UCLA School of Dentistry, Los Angeles, California

**LOUIS M. LIN, BDS, DMD, PhD**
Diplomate, American Board of Endodontics; Professor, Department of Endodontics, New York University College of Dentistry, New York, New York

**JUNQI LING, DDS, PhD**
Professor, Department of Operative Dentistry and Endodontics, Guanghua School of Stomatology, Hospital of Stomatology, Guangdong Province Key Laboratory of Stomatology, Sun Yat-sen University, Guangzhou, Guangdong, China

**YAO LIU, DDS, PhD**
Department of Anatomy and Cell Biology, School of Dental Medicine, University of Pennsylvania, Philadelphia, Pennsylvania; Department of Pediatric Dentistry, School of Stomatology, China Medical University, Shenyang, China

**SANJAY M. MALLYA, MDS, PhD**
Associate Professor; Residency Program Director; Section of Oral and Maxillofacial Radiology, UCLA School of Dentistry, Los Angeles, California

**JEREMY J. MAO, DDS, PhD**
Department of Operative Dentistry and Endodontics, Guanghua School of Stomatology, Hospital of Stomatology, Guangdong Province Key Laboratory of Stomatology, Sun Yat-sen University, Guangzhou, Guangdong, China; Professor and Edwin S. Robinson Endowed Chair; Director, Division of Endodontics, Center for Craniofacial Regeneration, Columbia University Medical Center, Columbia University, New York, New York

**XUELI MAO, DDS, PhD**
Department of Anatomy and Cell Biology, School of Dental Medicine, University of Pennsylvania, Philadelphia, Pennsylvania; Department of Operative Dentistry and Endodontics, Guanghua School of Stomatology, Hospital of Stomatology, Sun Yat-sen University, Guangzhou, Guangdong, China

**SHEBLI MEHRAZARIN, DDS, PhD**
Project Scientist, The Shapiro Family Laboratory of Viral Oncology and Aging Research, Section of Endodontics, UCLA School of Dentistry, Los Angeles, California

**ERIKA SALES JOVIANO PEREIRA, DDS, MS, PhD**
Department of Dental Clinic, School of Dentistry, Federal University of Bahia, Salvador, Bahia, Brazil

**OVE ANDREAS PETERS, DMD, MS, PhD**
Department of Endodontics, University of the Pacific Arthur A. Dugoni School of Dentistry, San Francisco, California

**NIKITA B. RUPAREL, MS, DDS, PhD**
Assistant Professor, Department of Endodontics, University of Texas Health Science Center at San Antonio, San Antonio, Texas

**SONGTAO SHI, DDS, PhD**
Department of Anatomy and Cell Biology, School of Dental Medicine, University of Pennsylvania, Philadelphia, Pennsylvania

**COLBY SMITH, DDS**
Section of Restorative Dentistry, UCLA School of Dentistry, Los Angeles, California

**SUHJIN SOHN, DDS, PhD**
The Shapiro Family Laboratory of Viral Oncology and Aging Research, UCLA School of Dentistry, Los Angeles, California

**MINJU SONG, DDS, PhD**
The Shapiro Family Laboratory of Viral Oncology and Aging Research; Section of Restorative Dentistry, UCLA School of Dentistry, Los Angeles, California

**RICHARD G. STEVENSON, DDS**
Section of Restorative Dentistry, UCLA School of Dentistry, Los Angeles, California

**BO YU, DDS, PhD**
Section of Restorative Dentistry, UCLA School of Dentistry, Los Angeles, California

**JUAN ZHONG, DDS**
Division of Endodontics, Center for Craniofacial Regeneration, Columbia University Medical Center, Columbia University, New York, New York

# Contents

teeth and immature teeth with an open apex. Besides these goals, the objectives of endodontic treatment of immature teeth include preservation of pulp vitality and often further root maturation. Robust criteria for outcome assessment are an essential determinant for any measure of treatment success for both mature and immature teeth.

## Modern Endodontic Microsurgery Concepts: A Clinical Update

Spyros Floratos and Syngcuk Kim

Increased use of the surgical operating microscope in endodontic surgery has elucidated many shortcomings of previous techniques and, along with microsurgical instruments and new more biologically acceptable root-end filling materials, has started the new microsurgical era in surgical endodontics. Endodontic microsurgery is a minimally invasive technique that results in less postoperative pain and edema and faster wound healing. It offers a significantly higher success rate than traditional apical surgery technique. The components, key concepts and procedural steps of endodontic microsurgery as well as the prognosis and predictability of modern root-end procedures are presented in this review.

## Clinical and Molecular Perspectives of Reparative Dentin Formation: Lessons Learned from Pulp-Capping Materials and the Emerging Roles of Calcium

Minju Song, Bo Yu, Sol Kim, Marc Hayashi, Colby Smith, Suhjin Sohn, Euiseong Kim, James Lim, Richard G. Stevenson, and Reuben H. Kim

The long-term use of calcium hydroxide and the recent increase in the use of hydraulic calcium-silicate cements as direct pulp-capping materials provide important clues in terms of how reparative dentin may be induced to form a "biological seal" to protect the underlying pulp tissues. In this review article, we discuss clinical and molecular perspectives of reparative dentin formation based on evidence learned from the use of these pulp-capping materials. We also discuss the emerging role of calcium as an odontoinductive component in these pulp-capping materials.

## Regenerative Endodontic Procedures: Clinical Outcomes

Anibal Diogenes and Nikita B. Ruparel

Immature teeth are at risk for pulp necrosis, resulting in arrested root development and poor long-term prognosis. There is growing evidence that regenerative endodontic procedures promote desirable clinical outcomes. Despite significant advances in the field of regenerative endodontics and acceptable clinical outcomes, current evidence suggests that the tissues formed following currently used procedures do not completely recapitulate the former pulp-dentin complex. Further research is needed to identify prognostic factors and predictors of successful outcomes and to develop different treatment strategies to better predictably achieve all 3 identified clinical outcomes, while favoring tissue formation that more closely resembles the pulp-dentin complex.

# DENTAL CLINICS OF NORTH AMERICA

**THE CLINICS ARE AVAILABLE ONLINE!**
Access your subscription at:
www.theclinics.com

# Preface

# Endodontics at the Verge of New Era Driven by Biological Innovation

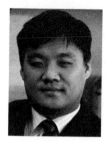

Mo K. Kang, DDS, PhD
*Editor*

Our field of Endodontics has undergone major transformations in the past decades in several fronts, including our basic understanding of the microbial cause, advances in biomechanical instrumentation of root canals, microsurgical techniques with predictable outcomes, and enhanced visibility using surgical microscopes. In addition, development of silicate-based cements, for example, mineral trioxide aggregate and bioceramics, which provide enhanced marginal seal with unsurpassed biocompatibility, now allows successful management of endodontic cases that have not been thought possible. Endodontics today enjoys the richness in technological advancements and accumulated evidence-based knowledge that guide our clinical principles and practices, leading to retention of more natural teeth than ever before. In this special issue of the *Dental Clinics of North America*, we present the state of our current knowledge at its pinnacle in contemporary Endodontics, including microbiology and pathogenesis of pulpal and periarticular diseases, innovations in root canal instrumentation, and the prognostic studies. As demonstrated in various articles of this issue, our level of understanding of the disease and ability to manage a diverse spectrum of Endodontic cases with predictable outcomes is remarkable.

Despite these successes, Endodontics today is faced with at least two discernible challenges. First, the prevalence of Endodontic pathoses, for example, apical periodontitis, in the general population is still very high, and it can be even higher in certain groups of individuals, such as the elderly population or those with previous root canal obturation with propensity for leakage. Hence, apical periodontitis continues to be the primary disease entity in Endodontics. One article in this issue deals with detailed molecular mechanisms of apical periodontitis as a disease model in Endodontics and includes discussion of our recent understanding of epigenetic regulators, which may regulate cellular responses to endodontic infection. Persistent postoperative apical

Dent Clin N Am 61 (2017) xi–xii
http://dx.doi.org/10.1016/j.cden.2016.09.001
0011-8532/17/© 2016 Published by Elsevier Inc.

**dental.theclinics.com**

periodontitis is a reflection of ongoing inflammatory signaling in response to bacterial infections in the root canal system. From histological studies, it is evident that bacterial irritants in infected root canals may reside in the areas, for example, isthmuses, lateral canals, and apical ramifications, that are not accessible to mechanical instrumentation or chemical debridement. Thus, a fundamental challenge in Endodontics is eradication of bacteria from the root canal system so as to reduce the prevalence of apical periodontitis. The second challenge is restoration of functional pulp in lieu of root canal filling materials. Besides sensibility through Aδ and C fibers, dental pulp provides critical defense mechanisms against microbial insults. Reparative dentin formation protects the pulp from eminent exposure to carious bacteria. Also, dental pulp is equipped with immune surveillance through dendritic cells at the pulp periphery as well as innate and adaptive immune responses that can surmount a massive attack on invading bacteria. In addition, dental pulp is ultimately engaged in root development by being the source of undifferentiated dental/apical papillae cells, which differentiate into functional odontoblasts. Sensibility in dental pulp also provides crucial protection of dentition from excessive changes in temperature, pressure, and caries. As such, restoration of normal pulp to function as part of endodontic therapies may be beneficial over root canal filling with inorganic materials.

After the discovery of mesenchymal stem cells (MSCs) in the dental pulp in 2000 by Dr Songtao Shi, stem cell research in Endodontics has expanded tremendously with a long-range goal of reinstituting functional dental pulp in teeth with pulpal necrosis. This goal is still on-going, but strides have been made in clinical Endodontics to incorporate regenerative procedures, for example, revascularization, in patient care. Three articles in this issue highlight the recent advances in clinical and translational aspects of on-going efforts in Regenerative Endodontics. Arguably, endodontic therapies harnessing pulp regeneration is one of the biggest things that happened in modern Endodontics and will continue to shape the future of our specialty. End-point in this endeavor may be regeneration of dental pulp to full function, which is clearly a step further from revascularization, and will require our understanding of neovascularization, neurogenesis, molecular mechanisms underlying pulpal immunology, inflammatory signaling, odontogenesis, and MSC biology in general. Pulp is fairly small tissue by size but mighty by the level of science enclosed within.

Mo K. Kang, DDS, PhD
Division of Constitutive and Regenerative Sciences
Section of Endodontics
UCLA School of Dentistry
CHS 43-007
10833 Le Conte Avenue
Los Angeles, CA 90095, USA

E-mail address:
mkang@dentistry.ucla.edu

# Endodontic Microbiology and Pathobiology
## Current State of Knowledge

Ashraf F. Fouad, DDS, MS

### KEYWORDS

- Endodontic microbiology • Immunology • Stem cells • Healing • Systemic diseases
- Genetic polymorphism

### KEY POINTS

- Greater microbial complexity has recently been revealed in endodontic infections.
- The host response–microbial interactions result in clinical presentation and response to healing.
- The host response is multifactorial and relates to many host factors and disease expression parameters.

### INTRODUCTION

Endodontic disease in the pulp or the periapex results from irritation by a complex array of microorganisms that normally populate the oral cavity. Despite being commensal under normal conditions, the composition of the microflora changes in the necrotic pulp, and many of the microorganisms involved increase in abundance and pathogenicity. The dental pulp, despite exhibiting a robust immunologic response, is clearly compromised in its ability to defend itself against advancing oral microflora, due to its lack of collateral circulation and its enclosure within the mineralized tissues of the tooth. Therefore, the pulp loses its vitality under these conditions at rates that are higher than any other tissue in the body, and a periapical lesion ensues. The periapical lesion has the fundamental biological function of prevention of the spread of infection that would result in osteonecrosis, osteomyelitis, and/or disseminating endodontic infections.

There is a large body of literature that describes the microbial irritants of the pulp and periapical tissues and the microbial-host interactions in these tissues. The intent of this review is to summarize recent advances in this area and provide a perspective

Disclosure Statement: The author has nothing to disclose.
Department of Endodontics, School of Dentistry, University of North Carolina at Chapel Hill, 1098 First Dental Building, CB# 7450, Chapel Hill, NC 27599-7450, USA
E-mail address: afouad@unc.edu

Dent Clin N Am 61 (2017) 1–15
http://dx.doi.org/10.1016/j.cden.2016.08.001
0011-8532/17/© 2016 Elsevier Inc. All rights reserved.

dental.theclinics.com

on the direction of new knowledge in this field, and its direct relationship to potential advances in clinical diagnosis, establishment of the prognosis, and biologically based treatment.

## CONTEMPORARY MICROBIOLOGICAL ANALYSIS

It has long been known that endodontic disease is fundamentally a microbial disease, and that rather than one or several bacterial or fungal species, the disease is initiated and propagated by a complex community of microorganisms that are common members of commensal oral microflora. **Table 1** summarizes the main advantages of different microbial detection methodologies. For decades, the gold standard was to culture bacteria (and to a lesser degree fungi) from infected root canals or periapical abscesses, in order to study their virulence, interactions, and susceptibilities to local and systemic treatment strategies. Although culturing remains the technique of choice for studying the phenotypic characteristics of bacteria and their susceptibility to antimicrobials, it has become clear recently that only about half of oral bacteria are cultivable[1] and that the oral cavity (and presumably the endodontic environment) contains many microorganisms that are not cultivable but may contribute to a significant degree in the pathogenesis of disease and resistance to treatment.[2] Moreover, some bacteria that are ordinarily readily cultivable in the oral environment may be rendered uncultivable despite being viable if the environment contains materials or conditions that interfere with growth in the laboratory. This is especially relevant in the endodontic environment, particularly if bacteria are exposed to some endodontic materials used during treatment and which may temporary interfere with bacterial growth, such as calcium hydroxide or antibiotics.[3,4]

**Table 1**
**Common methods of microbial identification and the information that each provides**

| Culturing | Imaging | Molecular Methods |
|---|---|---|
| Allows the study of microbial virulence | Allows accurate identification of location and density of microorganisms | High sensitivity of microbial detection |
| Allows testing of antibiotic resistance | Higher magnifications allow examination of different microbial forms, shapes and biofilm structure | Accurate taxonomic classification of microorganisms, identification of pathogenic strains, and relative abundance of different taxa |
| Allows in vitro testing and experimentation | Is useful for some fastidious organisms, such as spirochetes being observed with dark-field microscopy | Accurate study of microbial virulence, interactions, and gene expression |
| Easily identifies bacterial load (numbers) | Requires analysis of extracted teeth or smears from patients | Comprehensive analysis of protein expression; approximate estimation of bacterial load |
| Shows microbial viability | Vitality stains allow determination of live and dead forms | Viability can be confirmed with detection of mRNA |

Sampling the endodontic environment is also very challenging. It is well known that bacteria grow in the form of biofilm on root canal walls that form over weeks, months, or years depending on the age of the infection. Sampling using paper points placed in uninstrumented canal mainly captures planktonic bacteria. Even if files are used to disrupt the biofilm, the files are known to touch a small percentage of the canal wall surface area. Isthmi, fins, lateral canals, or dentinal tubules are rarely reached by sampling tools. The contribution of coronal and apical bacterial microflora to the pathogenesis, disease presentation, or resistance to healing is likely different. Therefore, sampling is likely to show a small proportion of root canal bacteria present, and methods that use imaging of bacteria in situ provide more accurate description of the bacterial presence.

Over the last 2 decades, significant advances have been made in molecular methods for microbial detection, identification, and enumeration. Molecular methods improve sensitivity (the ability to detect low levels of bacteria), accuracy of taxonomic classification, and depth of coverage. Different generations of molecular methods have been used, starting with specific amplification of a microbial species, to broad range cloning and sequencing of bacterial 16S gene to identify representatives of unknown bacteria present in the community, to the use of deep sequencing that allows the detection of a large proportion of bacteria, including low-abundance taxa.[5–7]

Contemporary microbiological analysis involves much more that the mere identification of the bacterial or fungal species present.[6] It is well known that specific strains of bacteria are more virulent than others, and that within a certain microbial composition and environment, bacteria of the same species may behave differently. In addition, bacteria may start to express important virulence genes when their numbers reach a certain threshold, a property referred to a quorum sensing.[8,9] Therefore, molecular microbiology currently exploits the widespread availability and reduced cost of sequencing to examine the genetic profiles of all bacteria present. This process, commonly referred to as metagenomic analysis or shotgun sequencing, allows the identification of a myriad of genes related to taxonomy, structure, function, virulence and antibiotic resistance.[10,11] Identifying the genes is insufficient to determine the function, as it only determines the potential for certain functionalities to be present. A more applied methodology involves an analysis of the actual bacterial (and host) proteins expressed or proteomic analysis,[12–14] or the metabolic pathways leading to specific activities or transcriptomics.[13,15]

## CLINICALLY RELEVANT MICROBIOLOGICAL FINDINGS

There are several ways in which the ability to detect bacteria, or identify specific microorganisms, in an endodontic case may be directly useful clinically. For example, the presence of residual bacteria at the time of obturation may be predictive of long-term outcomes; specific microorganisms may be associated with more symptomatic endodontic infections and with antibiotic resistance. The presence of viruses systemically or fungi locally may render the infections more aggressive and more difficult to treat.

Numerous studies have shown that the prognosis of endodontic treatment of cases with vital pulp is very high, and that the prognosis decreases by 15% to 20% in cases with preoperative infections.[16,17] Therefore, studies sought to determine if the presence of bacteria at the time of obturation may be a good indicator of long-term outcomes. Several studies did show this to be true,[18–20] although this was not universally found.[21] One elegant study done on primate models showed not only that residual bacteria can predict outcomes of endodontic treatment but also that the persistence of those bacteria at the time of follow-up was an even stronger predictor of results.[22]

Therefore, many studies have been performed to determine the efficacy of technologies used in root canal preparation and disinfection used the elimination of bacteria as a surrogate outcome for success of treatment. For example, it has been shown that ultrasonic irrigation of hypochlorite was more efficacious,[23] whereas passive ultrasonic activation,[24,25] passive sonic activation,[26] and apical negative pressure irrigation[27] were not more efficacious than controls in eliminating bacteria.

With respect to root canal instrumentation, nickel-titanium (NiTi) rotary instrumentation[28] and the self-adjusting file[29] were shown to be more efficacious than hand NiTi instruments. In addition, it was recently shown that rotary NiTi instrumentation was equivalent from a microbiological perspective to instrumentation activated by reciprocation.[30] All these studies were clinically performed on teeth with infections, and various methods of bacterial detection were used. One other study did not assess the microbiological status of the prepared canal, but examined several sizes of apical preparation in infected canals. The results showed significant improvement in healing when preparation was performed to 3 file sizes larger than the initial file, and a dose-response improved healing for larger apical sizes.[31] Given that all cases in this study had large canals with apical periodontitis, it is assumed that the larger sizes created more disruption of apical bacterial biofilm, and elimination of more bacteria through disinfectant irrigation.

Specific microorganisms may be associated with clinical symptoms of the patient. This hypothesis has been tested in numerous studies over the years. However, more recent data that use next generation sequencing show no specific patterns of association with symptoms.[32–34] Older studies proposed that symptoms may be related to the patients having certain types of systemic viral effects, such as human cytomegalovirus and Epstein-Barr virus.[35,36] However, more recent data could not confirm these findings,[37,38] and a recent systematic review showed no definitive associations of these viruses with symptoms,[39] although they were associated with diseased periapical tissues more significantly than normal pulp.[40] Fungi are present in about 10% to 25% of endodontic infections.[41–43] Their significance is that they express a variety of virulence factors, particularly in association with bacteria,[44] and are difficult to eradicate from the root canal environment.[45,46] Inadequate isolation of teeth during root canal treatment or leaving root canals open between appointments would increase the opportunity for fungi to populate the root canal environment.

As noted previously, there is a great amount of diversity in bacterial pathogens that are thought to contribute to endodontic disease. The sources of these microorganisms are those that normal inhabit the oral cavity, or specifically the gingival microflora. It has been observed that specific endodontic and periodontal pathogens correlate closely in their prevalence, in cases of endodontic and periodontal disease.[47] More recently, a study using contemporary sequencing methodologies showed that despite similarities in overall composition, there are differences in abundance of bacteria in root canal and periodontal environments of endodontic-periodontal lesions.[48] The study further revealed the changes in bacterial abundance after treatment of either condition (**Table 2**).

Therefore, during pathogenesis of endodontic infections, microbial irritants that are the forefront of the infection are the first among the large numbers of oral or periodontal microorganisms to reach the root canal and advance toward the periapical tissues. Eventually, ecological and nutritional pressures shape the resultant community to have many of the original taxa, albeit in different proportions. One study that examined the progression of bacteria from the normal oral environment to the necrotic root

**Table 2**
**Microbial abundance in the periodontal pockets and root canals of combined endodontic-periodontal lesions**

| Periodontal Preoperative | | Periodontal Postoperative | | Endodontic Preoperative | | Endodontic After Instrumentation | |
|---|---|---|---|---|---|---|---|
| Fusobacterium nucleatum ssp nucleatum[a] | 53 | Parvimonas micra[a] | 40 | Prevotella intermedia[a] | 67 | Fusobacterium nucleatum ssp nucleatum[a] | 73 |
| Prevotella intermedia[a] | 40 | Prevotella intermedia[a] | 33 | Fusobacterium nucleatum ssp nucleatum[a] | 54 | Enterococcus faecalis[c] | 46 |
| Streptococcus constellatus[a] | 40 | Desulfobulbus sp oral taxon 041[b] | 23 | Parvimonas micra[a] | 33 | Staphylococcus genus probe | 10 |
| Desulfobulbus sp oral taxon 041[b] | 18 | Streptococcus constellatus[a] | 20 | Enterococcus faecalis[c] | 22 | Prevotella intermedia[a] | 7 |
| Actinomyces israelii[a] | 13 | Enterococcus faecalis[c] | 20 | Enterococcus faecalis[a] | 20 | Streptococcus salivarius/vestibularis[a] | 7 |
| Streptococcus genus probe | 11 | Actinomyces israelii[a] | 13 | Parvimonas micra[c] | 15 | Actinomyces genus probe | 4 |
| Parvimonas micra[c] | 9 | Parvimonas micra[c] | 11 | Streptococcus constellatus[a] | 13 | Streptococcus genus probe | 4 |
| Enterococcus faecalis[c] | 7 | Porphyromonas gingivalis[a] | 9 | Streptococcus salivarius/vestibularis[a] | 13 | Streptococcus salivarius/vestibularis[c] | 2 |
| Fusobacterium genus probe | 4 | Streptococcus genus probe | 7 | Bacteroidaceae [G-1] sp oral taxon 272[c] | 5 | Fusobacterium genus probe | 2 |
| Streptococcus constellatus[c] | 3 | Fusobacterium genus probe | 4 | Stomatobaculum sp oral taxon 373[b] | 4 | Parvimonas micra[c] | 2 |
| | | Filifactor alocis[c] | 3 | Peptostreptococcaceae [13] [G-1] sp oral taxon 113[c] | 3 | Prevotella nigrescens[c] | 1 |

[a] Next Generation Sequencing.
[b] Phylotype.
[c] Culture.

*Adapted from* Gomes BP, Berber VB, Kokaras AS, et al. Microbiomes of endodontic-periodontal lesions before and after chemomechanical preparation. J Endod 2015;41(12):1975–84; with permission.

canal, to the periapical abscess, in the same group of patients showed the degree to which this overlap occurs[49] (**Fig. 1**). The data show the complexity of the microbial composition in different patients and provide a new dimension to the phrase "polymicrobial infections."

## ADVANCES IN RESEARCH ON HOST RESPONSE TO ENDODONTIC PATHOGENS

There is no doubt that the host response in the dental pulp or the periapical lesion is a major factor that shapes, modulates, and degrades the microbial irritants in these sites. The host response varies in different individuals, and this is one of the reasons for the complex microbial diversity discussed previously.

The immunologic response to pulpal and periapical irritation is orchestrated by a large number of cellular and molecular components with various functions and specificities (**Table 3**). Hundreds of these immunologic factors have been described in recent years, the discussion of which is beyond the scope of this review. The reader is referred to other more comprehensive reviews of the subject.[50] The emphasis in this review is on recent findings, especially those that may potentially have direct clinical relevance.

Older clinical studies have shown that several of these mediators are significantly associated with pain. For example, symptomatic irreversible pulpitis has been associated with significantly increased pulpal eicosanoids,[51] bradykinin,[52] and neuropeptides like substance P.[53] It was not clear, however, why these mediators were increased in certain patients, in a disease process that mimics histologically many other cases where the pulp is asymptomatic or mildly symptomatic. In the last decade, it was shown that trigeminal nociceptors have receptors for toll-like receptor-4 (TLR-4)

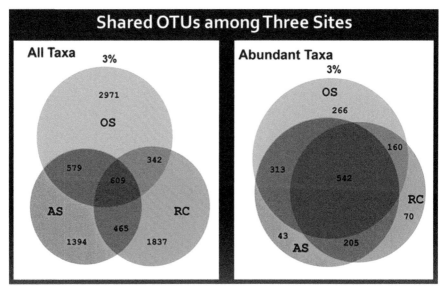

**Fig. 1.** The number of operational taxonomic units (OTUs) with shared similarities in the 16S gene of bacteria from 8 patients who had no oral disease except acute apical abscess in a tooth that had trauma or had deep restoration. The Venn diagrams represent the shared tax among the oral cavity (OS), necrotic root canal (RC), and apical abscess (AS). (*Adapted from* Hsiao WW, Li KL, Liu Z, et al. Microbial transformation from normal oral microbiota to acute endodontic infections. BMC Genomics 2012;13:345; with permission.)

**Table 3**
**Commonly identified immunologic cells and molecular mediators in pulpal and periapical disease**

| Cells of the Innate Immunity | Cells of the Specific (Adaptive) Immunity | Proinflammatory Mediators | Anti-inflammatory Mediators |
|---|---|---|---|
| Neutrophils | T-helper 1 | Cytokines (eg, IL-1, IL-6, TNF-α, IL-12, IFN-γ, and IL-17) | Cytokines (eg, IL-1Ra, IL-4, IL-5, IL-10, IL-13) |
| Monocytes/macrophages (M1 and M2) | T-helper 2 | Chemokines (eg, CXCL8 or IL-8, CCL2 or MCP-1, CCL5 or RANTES) | Growth factors (TGF-β, VEGF, PDGF, IGF) |
| Dendritic cells (myeloid or plasmacytoid) | T-helper 9 | | Tissue inhibitors of MMPs |
| NK cells | T-helper 17 | MMPs | Other protease inhibitors |
| Eosinophils | T-helper 22 | Fibrinolytic and kinin proteins | Coagulation proteins and fibrin |
| Basophils | T-regulatory | Complement | Glucocorticoids |
| Mast cells | T-cytotoxic | Pattern recognition receptors (Toll-like receptors, TLR-2 and TLR-4) or NOD-like receptors | Endogenous opiates |
| | T-suppressor | Neuropeptides (substance P, CGRP, neurokinins) | Superoxide dismutase |
| | B cells | Oxygen-derived free radicals | Osteoprotegrin |
| | Innate lymphoid cells | Signal transduction proteins (eg, MyD88) | Nitric oxide |
| | | Transcription factor (eg, NF-κB) | |
| | | Adhesion molecules (eg, integrins and selectins) | |
| | | Antibodies | |
| | | Eicosanoids (eg, PGE2) | |
| | | Nitric oxide | |
| | | Acute phase proteins (eg, C-reactive protein, serum amyloid A) | |

and thus may be sensitized by lipopolysaccharide (LPS), which is found in gram-negative bacterial cell wall.[54,55] This finding explains the many other studies that have found significant associations between the presence of LPS in deep caries, root canals, or periapical tissues and pain.[56–58]

Moreover, it was recently reported that gene polymorphism of cyclooxygenase-2 gene may be associated with postoperative pain following endodontic therapy.[59] This discovery shows how different individuals may respond differently to treatment (and presumably to the original pathologic irritants) despite having the same cause and disease process.

One of the most important advances in host response research over the past decade has been the realization that the recognition of, and defense against, microbial irritants is not merely the function of immune cells but also is a function of structural cells such as odontoblasts, osteoblasts, and endothelial cells. The odontoblast is a cell that appears to have numerous immunologic functions, such as the expression of TLRs (TLR-2 and TLR-4) for the recognition of bacterial cell wall molecules, interaction with dendritic cells, and secretion of chemokines like interleukin-8 (IL-8) and of defensins that have strong antimicrobial function.[60,61] Odontoblasts are, therefore, capable of initiating the immunologic cascade that leads to mounting an immune response, which has importance when regeneration of these cells from dental pulp stem cells is contemplated.

In addition to the presence of stem cells in the dental pulp, it has been revealed in recent years that dentin is a reservoir for several growth factors like transforming growth factor-β, vascular endothelial growth factor, and fibroblast growth factor.[62] These factors can easily be released from dentin using materials such as EDTA, calcium hydroxide, or mineral trioxide aggregate (MTA), in order to assist with regenerative procedures of dental tissues.

Given the overwhelming interest in saving the vital pulp through vital pulp therapy procedures in recent years, there is a continuous search for molecular mediators that would allow the clinical differentiation of reversible and irreversible pulpitis. Saving the vital pulp is especially important in cases where pain is not a significant factor. It is known, for example, that about 40% of cases of pulpitis proceed to pulp necrosis without pain,[63] and about 8% to 15% of teeth that receive crowns or other restorations will eventually need endodontic therapy.[64] Recently, it was revealed that matrix metalloproteinase-9 (MMP-9) and tissue inactivator of matrix metalloproteinases-1 (TIMP-1) were significantly elevated in cases of irreversible pulpitis compared with patients with reversible pulpitis or normal pulp, or those with irreversible pulpitis but on nonsteroidal anti-inflammatory drugs.[65] Another more comprehensive study was performed to compare irreversible pulpitis and normal pulp as well as the various disease states of the dental pulp, using genome-wide microarray analysis.[66] The results showed several upregulated genes that represent various cytokines, TLRs, collagen formation genes, and others, including MMP-9. These studies show promise that knowledge of important genetic variations associated with disease may assist with accurate chair-side diagnosis of pulpal disease in the future. In addition to sampling the pulp directly, sampling may also be done of the gingival crevicular fluid of the affected tooth, and comparing it to contralateral tooth.[67,68]

The interplay of osteoblasts and osteoclasts, a process that is highly regulated, is critical for both the pathogenesis of periapical lesions and their healing (**Fig. 2**). The process occurs normally as part of physiologic bone turnover, which is regulated by hormonal and nutritional factors. In addition, important biological modulators such as LPS and peptidoglycan influence the direction and degree of bone resorption, which is critical for the formation of the lesion and the assembly of the immunologic reaction.

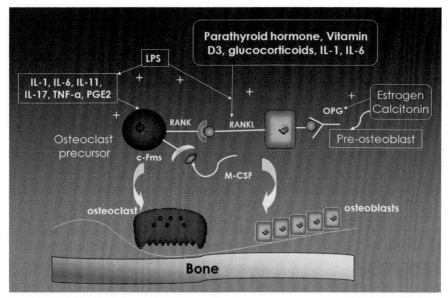

**Fig. 2.** Interactions between osteoblastic cells and osteoclast precursors during bone remodeling. PGE2, prostaglandin E2. (*Modified from* Rosen CJ, Bilezikian JP. Clinical review 123: anabolic therapy for osteoporosis. J Clin Endocrinol Metab 2001;86(3):957–64; and Boyle WJ, Simonet WS, Lacey DL. Osteoclast differentiation and activation. Nature 2003;423(6937):337–42; with permission.)

Studies have shown that apical bone resorption occurs concomitantly with progressive inflammation in the pulp[69] and can be seen radiographically using cone beam computed tomography in about 13% of pulpitis cases.[70] As the pulp degenerates and bacterial pathogens populate this space, larger periapical radiolucencies develop and encroach on the inner cortical plates of the mandible or maxilla, which give rise to the apical radiolucencies typically seen in association with necrotic pulp on periapical radiographs. Although the development of these radiographic lesions is relatively rapid,[71] complete healing usually takes months to years[16,17,19] and may take decades.[72,73]

Changes in the presence and size of the periapical lesions are thought to be fundamentally related to the presence or persistence of microbial irritants. Although cases with primary infections can be easily identified and treated, the situation in cases with preexisting endodontic treatment are more difficult to discern, particularly if the history of treatment is not available. Therefore, it is very difficult clinically to determine if a periapical lesion in these situations is healing, developing, or stable and to make a treatment decision accordingly. Recently, investigators have sought to measure certain mediators of bone resorption in periapical lesions, to gain insight into this issue. One study compared 83 granulomas retrieved surgically with 24 normal periodontal ligament samples. In this study,[74] it was decided to arbitrarily dichotomize the lesions using a threshold of 5-fold or greater ratio of RANKL to OPG for active lesions (more bone resorption) and the rest inactive lesions (or controls) (see **Fig. 2**). The study analyzed the expression of 84 wound-healing genes in active and inactive lesions. The results are shown in **Table 4**.

More recently, the same group analyzed periapical tissue fluid (sampling through the canal) for several MMPs and their inhibitors and found that MMP-2, MMP-7, and

**Table 4**
**Results on active/inactive lesions of 83 periapical granulomas based on RANKL/OPG ratio**

| Active Lesions | Inactive Lesions |
|---|---|
| TNF (cytokine) | SERPINE1 (remodeling enzyme) |
| CXCL11 (chemokine) | TIMP1 (remodeling enzyme) |
| | COL1A1 (ECM component) |
| | TGFB1 (growth factor) |
| | ITGA4 (cellular adhesion) |

*Adapted from* Garlet GP, Horwat R, Ray HL Jr, et al. Expression analysis of wound healing genes in human periapical granulomas of progressive and stable nature. J Endod 2012;38(2):185–90; with permission.

MMP-9 were significantly associated with a diagnosis of chronic apical abscess, whereas TIMP-1 was significantly associated with asymptomatic apical periodontitis.[75]

Clearly, bone resorption and deposition in the periapical area can be influenced by systemic diseases or medications that the patient may be taking. Studies have shown that pathogenesis and/or healing of periapical lesions may be related to diabetes mellitus,[76–78] sickle cell anemia,[79–81] and smoking.[82–84] Likewise, preliminary animal studies have shown that the pathogenesis of periapical lesions is affected by intravenous bisphosphonates,[85,86] statins,[87–89] and metformin (a drug used to treat diabetes mellitus type 2).[90]

## INDIVIDUALIZED PROGNOSIS OR PERSONALIZED ENDODONTICS

In the last 2 decades or so, studies have shown that gene polymorphism may occur among individuals leading to differences in disease susceptibility, clinical presentation, and response to therapy. Gene polymorphism is typically identified by detecting individual variation in gene sequences, as little as single-nucleotide polymorphism. As noted before, genetic polymorphism among patients may result in differences among them in disease expression and pain experience following endodontic treatment. In addition, several studies have now been performed, in which candidate genes have been examined for the effects that they may have on healing of endodontic disease 1 year after treatment, while controlling for other variables. Thus far, the research has shown that IL-β allele 2,[91] the FcγRIIA allele H131, and a combination of this allele with allele NA2 of the FcγRIIIB gene[92] were significantly linked to the healing status at 1 year in these studies. The role of IL-1β in bone resorption has been known for decades. The role of FcγR in healing is novel and less intuitive, because this receptor (commonly present on monocytes and macrophages) is associated with binding the Fc portion of the antibody molecule, thus helping with opsonization of antigens before phagocytosis.

In addition to gene polymorphisms, which relate to actual DNA differences, there are several epigenetic differences among patients that may also be operational in pathogenesis, disease expression, and healing. These epigenetic variations may relate to the degree of DNA methylation of the gene, or expression of noncoding small RNA molecules that influence gene expression. The available information shows that epigenetic differences may influence the expression of inflammatory mediators in pulpal and periapical tissues.[93–95] More data from large, well-controlled studies will be needed before these differences among patients can be used for diagnosis, the assessment of prognosis, or the determination of the treatment plan.

## REFERENCES

1. Paster BJ, Boches SK, Galvin JL, et al. Bacterial diversity in human subgingival plaque. J Bacteriol 2001;183(12):3770–83.

2. Siqueira JF Jr, Rocas IN. Uncultivated phylotypes and newly named species associated with primary and persistent endodontic infections. J Clin Microbiol 2005;43(7):3314–9.

3. Weiger R, de Lucena J, Decker HE, et al. Vitality status of microorganisms in infected human root dentine. Int Endod J 2002;35(2):166–71.

4. Fouad AF, Barry J. The effect of antibiotics and endodontic antimicrobials on the polymerase chain reaction. J Endod 2005;31(7):510–3.

5. Li L, Hsiao WW, Nandakumar R, et al. Analyzing endodontic infections by deep coverage pyrosequencing. J Dent Res 2010;89(9):980–4.

6. Siqueira JF Jr, Fouad AF, Rocas IN. Pyrosequencing as a tool for better understanding of human microbiomes. J Oral Microbiol 2012;4:1–15.

7. Fouad AF, Barry J, Caimano M, et al. PCR-based identification of bacteria associated with endodontic infections. J Clin Microbiol 2002;40(9):3223–31.

8. Wang BY, Alvarez P, Hong J, et al. Periodontal pathogens interfere with quorum-sensing-dependent virulence properties in Streptococcus mutans. J Periodontal Res 2011;46(1):105–10.

9. Siqueira JF Jr, Rôças IN. Community as the unit of pathogenicity: an emerging concept as to the microbial pathogenesis of apical periodontitis. Oral Surg Oral Med Oral Pathol Oral Radiol Endod 2009;107(6):870–8.

10. Siqueira JF Jr, Rocas IN. The oral microbiota: general overview, taxonomy, and nucleic acid techniques. Methods Mol Biol 2010;666:55–69.

11. Zehnder M, Belibasakis GN. On the dynamics of root canal infections—what we understand and what we don't. Virulence 2015;6(3):216–22.

12. Nandakumar R, Madayiputhiya N, Fouad AF. Proteomic analysis of endodontic infections by liquid chromatography-tandem mass spectrometry. Oral Microbiol Immunol 2009;24(4):347–52.

13. Paakkonen V, Tjaderhane L. High-throughput gene and protein expression analysis in pulp biologic research: review. J Endod 2010;36(2):179–89.

14. Provenzano JC, Siqueira JF Jr, Rôças IN, et al. Metaproteome analysis of endodontic infections in association with different clinical conditions. PLoS One 2013;8(10):e76108.

15. Liu C, Niu Y, Zhou X, et al. Streptococcus mutans copes with heat stress by multiple transcriptional regulons modulating virulence and energy metabolism. Sci Rep 2015;5:12929.

16. Ricucci D, Russo J, Rutberg M, et al. A prospective cohort study of endodontic treatments of 1,369 root canals: results after 5 years. Oral Surg Oral Med Oral Pathol Oral Radiol Endod 2011;112(6):825–42.

17. Ng YL, Mann V, Gulabivala K. A prospective study of the factors affecting outcomes of nonsurgical root canal treatment: part 1: periapical health. Int Endod J 2011;44(7):583–609.

18. Sundqvist G, Figdor D, Persson S, et al. Microbiologic analysis of teeth with failed endodontic treatment and the outcome of conservative re-treatment. Oral Surg Oral Med Oral Pathol Oral Radiol Endod 1998;85(1):86–93.

19. Sjogren U, Figdor D, Persson S, et al. Influence of infection at the time of root filling on the outcome of endodontic treatment of teeth with apical periodontitis. Int Endod J 1997;30(5):297–306.

20. Waltimo T, Trope M, Haapasalo M, et al. Clinical efficacy of treatment procedures in endodontic infection control and one year follow-up of periapical healing. J Endod 2005;31(12):863–6.

21. Peters LB, Wesselink PR. Periapical healing of endodontically treated teeth in one and two visits obturated in the presence or absence of detectable microorganisms. Int Endod J 2002;35(8):660–7.
22. Fabricius L, Dahlen G, Sundqvist G, et al. Influence of residual bacteria on periapical tissue healing after chemomechanical treatment and root filling of experimentally infected monkey teeth. Eur J Oral Sci 2006;114(4):278–85.
23. Burleson A, Nusstein J, Reader A, et al. The in vivo evaluation of hand/rotary/ultrasound instrumentation in necrotic, human mandibular molars. J Endod 2007;33(7):782–7.
24. Beus C, Safavi K, Stratton J, et al. Comparison of the effect of two endodontic irrigation protocols on the elimination of bacteria from root canal system: a prospective, randomized clinical trial. J Endod 2012;38(11):1479–83.
25. Paiva SS, Siqueira JF Jr, Rocas IN, et al. Molecular microbiological evaluation of passive ultrasonic activation as a supplementary disinfecting step: a clinical study. J Endod 2013;39(2):190–4.
26. Huffaker SK, Safavi K, Spangberg LS, et al. Influence of a passive sonic irrigation system on the elimination of bacteria from root canal systems: a clinical study. J Endod 2010;36(8):1315–8.
27. Pawar R, Alqaied A, Safavi K, et al. Influence of an apical negative pressure irrigation system on bacterial elimination during endodontic therapy: a prospective randomized clinical study. J Endod 2012;38(9):1177–81.
28. Rocas IN, Lima KC, Siqueira JF Jr. Reduction in bacterial counts in infected root canals after rotary or hand nickel-titanium instrumentation–a clinical study. Int Endod J 2013;46(7):681–7.
29. Neves MA, Rocas IN, Siqueira JF Jr. Clinical antibacterial effectiveness of the self-adjusting file system. Int Endod J 2014;47(4):356–65.
30. Neves MA, Provenzano JC, Rocas IN, et al. Clinical antibacterial effectiveness of root canal preparation with reciprocating single-instrument or continuously rotating multi-instrument systems. J Endod 2016;42(1):25–9.
31. Saini HR, Tewari S, Sangwan P, et al. Effect of different apical preparation sizes on outcome of primary endodontic treatment: a randomized controlled trial. J Endod 2012;38(10):1309–15.
32. Anderson AC, Al-Ahmad A, Elamin F, et al. Comparison of the bacterial composition and structure in symptomatic and asymptomatic endodontic infections associated with root-filled teeth using pyrosequencing. PLoS One 2013;8(12):e84960.
33. Saber MH, Schwarzberg K, Alonaizan FA, et al. Bacterial flora of dental periradicular lesions analyzed by the 454-pyrosequencing technology. J Endod 2012;38(11):1484–8.
34. Santos AL, Siqueira JF Jr, Rôças IN, et al. Comparing the bacterial diversity of acute and chronic dental root canal infections. PLoS One 2011;6(11):e28088.
35. Slots J, Nowzari H, Sabeti M. Cytomegalovirus infection in symptomatic periapical pathosis. Int Endod J 2004;37(8):519–24.
36. Yazdi KA, Sabeti M, Jabalameli F, et al. Relationship between human cytomegalovirus transcription and symptomatic apical periodontitis in Iran. Oral Microbiol Immunol 2008;23(6):510–4.
37. Chen V, Chen Y, Li H, et al. Herpesviruses in abscesses and cellulitis of endodontic origin. J Endod 2009;35(2):182–8.
38. Li H, Chen V, Chen Y, et al. Herpesviruses in endodontic pathoses: association of Epstein-Barr virus with irreversible pulpitis and apical periodontitis. J Endod 2009;35(1):23–9.

39. Jakovljevic A, Andric M. Human cytomegalovirus and Epstein-Barr virus in etio-pathogenesis of apical periodontitis: a systematic review. J Endod 2014;40(1): 6–15.

40. Jakovljevic A, Andric M, Knezevic A, et al. Human cytomegalovirus and Epstein-Barr virus genotypes in apical periodontitis lesions. J Endod 2015;41(11): 1847–51.

41. Waltimo TM, Siren EK, Torkko HL, et al. Fungi in therapy-resistant apical periodontitis. Int Endod J 1997;30(2):96–101.

42. Baumgartner JC, Watts CM, Xia T. Occurrence of Candida albicans in infections of endodontic origin. J Endod 2000;26(12):695–8.

43. Miranda TT, Vianna CR, Rodrigues L, et al. Diversity and frequency of yeasts from the dorsum of the tongue and necrotic root canals associated with primary apical periodontitis. Int Endod J 2009;42(9):839–44.

44. Miranda TT, Vianna CR, Rodrigues L, et al. Differential proteinase patterns among candida albicans strains isolated from root canal and lingual dorsum: possible roles in periapical disease. J Endod 2015;41(6):841–5.

45. Sen BH, Chugal NM, Liu H, et al. A new method for studying the adhesion of Candida albicans to dentin in the presence or absence of smear layer. Oral Surg Oral Med Oral Pathol Oral Radiol Endod 2003;96(2):201–6.

46. Siqueira JF Jr, Sen BH. Fungi in endodontic infections. Oral Surg Oral Med Oral Pathol Oral Radiol Endod 2004;97(5):632–41.

47. Rupf S, Kannengiesser S, Merte K, et al. Comparison of profiles of key periodontal pathogens in periodontium and endodontium. Endod Dent Traumatol 2000;16(6):269–75.

48. Gomes BP, Berber VB, Kokaras AS, et al. Microbiomes of endodontic-periodontal lesions before and after chemomechanical preparation. J Endod 2015;41(12): 1975–84.

49. Hsiao WW, Li KL, Liu Z, et al. Microbial transformation from normal oral microbiota to acute endodontic infections. BMC Genomics 2012;13:345.

50. Fouad AF, Huang GT-J. Inflammation and immunological responses. In: Rotstein I, editor. Ingle's endodontics. Chapter 9. 7th edition. Elsevier; 2016.

51. Cohen JS, Reader A, Fertel R, et al. A radioimmunoassay determination of the concentrations of prostaglandins E2 and F2alpha in painful and asymptomatic human dental pulps. J Endod 1985;11(8):330–5.

52. Lepinski AM, Hargreaves KM, Goodis HE, et al. Bradykinin levels in dental pulp by microdialysis. J Endod 2000;26(12):744–7.

53. Bowles WR, Withrow JC, Lepinski AM, et al. Tissue levels of immunoreactive substance P are increased in patients with irreversible pulpitis. J Endod 2003;29(4): 265–7.

54. Diogenes A, Ferraz CC, Akopian AN, et al. LPS sensitizes TRPV1 via activation of TLR4 in trigeminal sensory neurons. J Dent Res 2011;90(6):759–64.

55. Wadachi R, Hargreaves KM. Trigeminal nociceptors express TLR-4 and CD14: a mechanism for pain due to infection. J Dent Res 2006;85(1):49–53.

56. Yamasaki M, Nakane A, Kumazawa M, et al. Endotoxin and gram-negative bacteria in the rat periapical lesions. J Endod 1992;18(10):501–4.

57. Rocas IN, Lima KC, Assuncao IV, et al. Advanced caries microbiota in teeth with irreversible pulpitis. J Endod 2015;41(9):1450–5.

58. Jacinto RC, Gomes BP, Shah HN, et al. Quantification of endotoxins in necrotic root canals from symptomatic and asymptomatic teeth. J Med Microbiol 2005; 54(Pt 8):777–83.

59. Applebaum E, Nackley AG, Bair E, et al. Genetic variants in cyclooxygenase-2 contribute to post-treatment pain among endodontic patients. J Endod 2015; 41(8):1214–8.
60. Horst OV, Horst JA, Samudrala R, et al. Caries induced cytokine network in the odontoblast layer of human teeth. BMC Immunol 2011;12:9.
61. Horst OV, Tompkins KA, Coats SR, et al. TGF-beta1 inhibits TLR-mediated odontoblast responses to oral bacteria. J Dent Res 2009;88(4):333–8.
62. Smith AJ, Duncan HF, Diogenes A, et al. Exploiting the bioactive properties of the dentin-pulp complex in regenerative endodontics. J Endod 2016;42(1):47–56.
63. Michaelson PL, Holland GR. Is pulpitis painful? Int Endod J 2002;35(10):829–32.
64. Martin JA, Bader JD. Five-year treatment outcomes for teeth with large amalgams and crowns. Oper Dent 1997;22(2):72–8.
65. Mente J, Petrovic J, Gehrig H, et al. A prospective clinical pilot study on the level of matrix metalloproteinase-9 in dental pulpal blood as a marker for the state of inflammation in the pulp tissue. J Endod 2016;42(2):190–7.
66. Galicia JC, Henson BR, Parker JS, et al. Gene expression profile of pulpitis. Genes Immun 2016;17:239–43.
67. Awawdeh L, Lundy FT, Shaw C, et al. Quantitative analysis of substance P, neurokinin A and calcitonin gene-related peptide in pulp tissue from painful and healthy human teeth. Int Endod J 2002;35(1):30–6.
68. Awawdeh LA, Lundy FT, Linden GJ, et al. Quantitative analysis of substance P, neurokinin A and calcitonin gene-related peptide in gingival crevicular fluid associated with painful human teeth. Eur J Oral Sci 2002;110(3):185–91.
69. Fouad AF. IL-1 alpha and TNF-alpha expression in early periapical lesions of normal and immunodeficient mice. J Dent Res 1997;76(9):1548–54.
70. Abella F, Patel S, Duran-Sindreu F, et al. Evaluating the periapical status of teeth with irreversible pulpitis by using cone-beam computed tomography scanning and periapical radiographs. J Endod 2012;38(12):1588–91.
71. Fouad AF, Walton RE, Rittman BR. Induced periapical lesions in ferret canines: histologic and radiographic evaluation. Endod Dent Traumatol 1992;8(2):56–62.
72. Molven O, Halse A, Fristad I, et al. Periapical changes following root-canal treatment observed 20-27 years postoperatively. Int Endod J 2002;35(9):784–90.
73. Fristad I, Molven O, Halse A. Nonsurgically retreated root filled teeth–radiographic findings after 20-27 years. Int Endod J 2004;37(1):12–8.
74. Garlet GP, Horwat R, Ray HL Jr, et al. Expression analysis of wound healing genes in human periapical granulomas of progressive and stable nature. J Endod 2012;38(2):185–90.
75. Letra A, Ghaneh G, Zhao M, et al. MMP-7 and TIMP-1, new targets in predicting poor wound healing in apical periodontitis. J Endod 2013;39(9):1141–6.
76. Fouad AF, Burleson J. The effect of diabetes mellitus on endodontic treatment outcome: data from an electronic patient record. J Am Dent Assoc 2003; 134(1):43–51 [quiz: 117–8].
77. Fouad AF, Barry J, Russo J, et al. Periapical lesion progression with controlled microbial inoculation in a type I diabetic mouse model. J Endod 2002;28(1):8–16.
78. Garber SE, Shabahang S, Escher AP, et al. The effect of hyperglycemia on pulpal healing in rats. J Endod 2009;35(1):60–2.
79. Demirbaş Kaya A, Aktener BO, Unsal C. Pulpal necrosis with sickle cell anaemia. Int Endod J 2004;37(9):602–6.
80. Costa CP, Thomaz EB, Souza Sde F. Association between sickle cell anemia and pulp necrosis. J Endod 2013;39(2):177–81.

81. Ferreira SB, de Brito LC, Oliveira MP, et al. Periapical cytokine expression in sickle cell disease. J Endod 2015;41(3):358–62.
82. Krall EA, Abreu Sosa C, Garcia C, et al. Cigarette smoking increases the risk of root canal treatment. J Dent Res 2006;85(4):313–7.
83. Lopez-Lopez J, Jane-Salas E, Martin-Gonzalez J, et al. Tobacco smoking and radiographic periapical status: a retrospective case-control study. J Endod 2012;38(5):584–8.
84. Celeste RK, Gomes MS. Association between apical periodontitis and smoking. J Endod 2013;39(2):157.
85. Xiong H, Wei L, Hu Y, et al. Effect of alendronate on alveolar bone resorption and angiogenesis in rats with experimental periapical lesions. Int Endod J 2010;43(6): 485–91.
86. Kang B, Cheong S, Chaichanasakul T, et al. Periapical disease and bisphosphonates induce osteonecrosis of the jaws in mice. J Bone Miner Res 2013;28(7): 1631–40.
87. Lai EH, Hong CY, Kok SH, et al. Simvastatin alleviates the progression of periapical lesions by modulating autophagy and apoptosis in osteoblasts. J Endod 2012;38(6):757–63.
88. Lin LD, Lin SK, Chao YL, et al. Simvastatin suppresses osteoblastic expression of Cyr61 and progression of apical periodontitis through enhancement of the transcription factor Forkhead/winged helix box protein O3a. J Endod 2013;39(5): 619–25.
89. Shadmehr E, Khademi A. Effect of simvastatin on kinetics of osteoprotegrin/receptor activator nuclear kappa B Ligand mRNA expression in periapical lesions. Int Endod J 2013;46(11):1077–82.
90. Liu L, Zhang C, Hu Y, et al. Protective effect of metformin on periapical lesions in rats by decreasing the ratio of receptor activator of nuclear factor kappa B ligand/ osteoprotegerin. J Endod 2012;38(7):943–7.
91. Morsani JM, Aminoshariae A, Han YW, et al. Genetic predisposition to persistent apical periodontitis. J Endod 2011;37(4):455–9.
92. Siqueira JF Jr, Rôças IN, Provenzano JC, et al. Relationship between Fcgamma receptor and interleukin-1 gene polymorphisms and post-treatment apical periodontitis. J Endod 2009;35(9):1186–92.
93. Campos K, Gomes CC, de Fatima Correia-Silva J, et al. Methylation pattern of IFNG in periapical granulomas and radicular cysts. J Endod 2013;39(4):493–6.
94. Campos K, Gomes CC, Farias LC, et al. DNA methylation of MMP9 is associated with high levels of MMP-9 messenger RNA in periapical inflammatory lesions. J Endod 2016;42(1):127–30.
95. Cardoso FP, Viana MB, Sobrinho AP, et al. Methylation pattern of the IFN-gamma gene in human dental pulp. J Endod 2010;36(4):642–6.

# Molecular Mechanisms of Apical Periodontitis

## Emerging Role of Epigenetic Regulators

Shebli Mehrazarin, DDS, PhD[a], Abdullah Alshaikh, DDS[a],
Mo K. Kang, DDS, PhD[a,b],*

## KEYWORDS

- Apical periodontitis • Epigenetics • Histone methyltransferase
- Histone demethylase • Gene expression

## KEY POINTS

- Conventional endodontic therapies yield highly successful outcome, owing to efforts in enhanced diagnostic tool, antimicrobial therapeutics, and advances in biomaterials research. However, persistence in apical periodontitis (AP) in some cases presents with treatment challenges and necessitates further investigation of the molecular mechanisms underlying AP in order to innovate new therapeutic approaches.
- Earlier studies elucidated the role of inflammatory cytokines and intracellular signaling, for example, JAK/STAT pathway, leading to bone destruction associated with AP, and these research efforts were fueled by the availability of murine pulp exposure models with specific gene knockouts.
- "Epigenetics" refers to the mechanism of gene regulation through chromatin structure rather than changes in DNA nucleotide sequence. Recent studies have uncovered the role of epigenetic modulators, for example, histone Lys-specific methyltransferases (KMTs) and histone Lys-specific demethylases (KDMs), in gene regulation through altering the methylation status of histone tails, which may have permissive or restrictive roles in gene expression.
- Jmjd3, a KDM specific for trimethylated Lys 27 of histone 3 (H3K27Me3), regulates a multitude of target genes involved in diverse biological processes, including inflammatory signaling.

*Continued*

Disclosure: The authors disclose no conflict of interest.
[a] The Shapiro Family Laboratory of Viral Oncology and Aging Research, UCLA School of Dentistry, CHS 43-033, 10833 Le Conte Avenue, Los Angeles, CA 90095, USA; [b] Section of Endodontics, Division of Constitutive and Regenerative Sciences, UCLA School of Dentistry, CHS 43-007, 10833 Le Conte Avenue, Los Angeles, CA 90095, USA
* Corresponding address.
*E-mail address:* mkang@dentistry.ucla.edu

Dent Clin N Am 61 (2017) 17–35
http://dx.doi.org/10.1016/j.cden.2016.08.003
0011-8532/17/© 2016 Published by Elsevier Inc.

dental.theclinics.com

*Continued*

- Structure-based drug screening identified selective inhibitor of Jmjd3, GSK-J1/J4, which demonstrate anti-inflammatory effects by suppressing tumor necrosis factor-$\alpha$ expression in lipopolysaccharide-activated human macrophages. Future research should focus on the regulatory molecules of AP to innovate novel therapeutic approaches.

## INTRODUCTION

The efficacy of conventional root canal therapies (RCTs) has been the subject of numerous studies at different levels of evidence in part because of the number of patients and teeth that are affected by pulpal infection. In the United States alone, approximately 15 million RCTs are performed annually (www.aae.org), which may surmount to dental care cost of more than $10 billion per year. Several studies, dating back to 1956 published by Strindberg,[1] and more recent studies with contemporary healing criteria, indicate that RCTs demonstrate highly efficacious outcome exceeds 90% healing rates.[2–4] On the contrary, several cross-sectional studies demonstrate quite alarming numbers in the occurrence of apical periodontitis (AP), when detected by common periapical radiographs. For instance, AP occurred in 27% of general population in Finland with 39% associated with endodontically treated teeth as opposed to 9% in untreated teeth.[5] In another study, AP was found in 40% of teeth with prior endodontic treatments.[6] In a large cross-sectional study examining 1030 endodontically treated teeth, Song and colleagues[7] reported 43.7% incidence of radiographic AP in teeth with inadequate endodontic treatment, whereas those with adequate endodontic treatment were found diseased at 17.7%, given acceptable coronal restoration. When both endodontic treatment and coronal restoration were compromised, the incidence of AP was found at 58.8%. Although the cross-sectional studies have limitations in distinguishing between diseased periapical state from those undergoing healing process after endodontic treatment, the sheer number of radiographically detectable AP in the general population is quite alarming and do warrant further investigation as to whether the treatment success is inflated in some studies, and whether treatment modalities can be improved to reduce the occurrence of AP in the general population.

A systematic review of published outcomes studies reported a wide range of treatment outcomes from 31% to 96% for primary endodontic cases reviewed in papers published from 1922 to 2002,[8] indicating a number of compounding variables that affect the treatment outcomes emphasized in different studies. In almost all outcomes studies, one of the most significant prognostic factors is the presence or absence of AP. As illustrated by Sjogren and colleagues,[9] Endodontic treatment resulted in the outcomes of 96% and 86% in the cases without and with AP, respectively. Treatment outcome is further compromised at 62% for re-treatment cases presenting with AP. Similarly, Marquis and colleagues[4] reported 93% success rate for primary endodontic cases without AP and reduced 80% for the cases presented with AP. When the outcomes assessment is performed by cone-beam computed tomography, the presence of AP upon recall was detected at 25.9%, whereas AP was noted in 12.6% of cases reviewed by conventional periapical radiographs.[10] As such, endodontic treatment outcome cannot be described by a singular number because it is greatly affected by multiple contributing factors, among which the presence of AP appears to be predominating.

Endodontic pathoses with or without AP are in fact vastly different disease entities requiring different treatment approaches. Because the presence and extent of AP are linked to microbial infection of the root canal system,[11] endodontic treatment of cases with AP should focus on antimicrobial modalities, be it instrumentation, chemome-chanical debridement, or intracanal medicaments. On the contrary, the cases with vital pulp without AP lack microbial infection in the root canals; conventional root canal therapies (cRCT) for such cases are essentially palliative and preventive against future microbial infection of the root canal system. This fundamental distinction between the endodontic pathoses with or without AP explains the difference in the treatment outcomes. AP is routinely detected by periapical radiographs due to alveolar bone destruction at the site of inflammation, which primarily involves apical ramifications of infected root canals. Anatomic variations at the apical ramifications could drastically complicate the endodontic treatment outcomes for cases with AP. For instance, 86% of mandibular first molars contain 2 mesial canals and isthmus, and 70% of these teeth contain isthmus at within 2 mm from the root apex.[12] Also, 31% of maxillary molars possess 2 mesial canals connected through complete isthmus to root apex.[13] Histo-logic study showed that established biofilm in isthmi cannot be removed by root canal instrumentation, allowing for persistent AP.[14] Also, the importance of extraradicular infection in posttreatment AP has been reported by several studies. Extraradicular infection is often associated with specific bacterial species, for example, *Actinomyces isralii*, forming apical actinomycoses, but others reported extraradicular coagulation of multiple bacterial genera, for example, *Prevotella*, *Streptococcus*, and *Fusobacterium*, in acute endodontic abscess, or in the form of apical calculus, causing persistent AP.[15–19] Therefore, AP is a unique subset of endodontic pathoses contributed by persistent microbial infection of the root canals and should really be distinguished from pulpitis in the understanding of pathogenesis, therapeutic modalities, and outcomes assessment.

In addition to local tissue destructive effects, several studies demonstrate possible linkage between AP and systemic conditions, such as cardiovascular diseases, diabetes, and preterm birth. In a recent study, An and colleagues[20] reported that radiographically diagnosed AP in 182 patients was associated with increased incidence of cardiovascular accident and hypercholesterolemia against an equal number of aged- and gender-matched control patients with AP. Likewise, earlier studies uncovered chronic periodontal infection as a risk factor for systemic diseases, like atherosclerosis and pulmonary diseases.[21,22] At a mechanistic level, intraoral inoculation of periodontal pathogens in susceptible mice (eg, deficiency of integrin β6) led to increased periodontal bone loss, increased infiltration of the bacteria into aortic vasculature, and increased size of atherosclerotic plaque compared with normal control mice.[23] Inasmuch as AP can be silently present in patients at high incidence,[5–7] AP still poses significant risk in systemic health in addition to local tissue destruction associated with persistent root canal infection. Mechanistic understanding of AP is of paramount importance in innovating effective means of diagnosis and therapeutics.

Earlier studies established animal models of AP associated with root canal infection by intentional pulp exposure to the oral cavity,[24,25] and use of genetically altered mice provided unique experimental tools with which to study inflammatory signaling from AP.[26,27] Although these earlier studies identified these effector molecules, for example, cytokines and inflammatory signaling molecules, of periapical inflammation, the mechanisms leading to their regulation and response to inflammatory signaling are well understood. Recent studies reported the role of the epigenetic regulators in diverse biological functions, including inflammation and immune regulation.[28,29] In this review, the current understanding of the mechanisms of AP, the concept of epigenetic gene regulation, and mechanisms by which epigenetic modulators determine inflammatory signaling through target gene regulation are discussed.

## BASIC DISEASE MECHANISMS OF APICAL PERIODONTITIS AND PREDISPOSING FACTORS

AP is an inflammatory disease that results in significant bone and tissue destruction. It involves accumulation of oral bacteria that play an important role in initiating and sustaining infection and inflammation within periapical lesions. Although endodontic pathoses, like others in the oral cavity, result from polymicrobial infection, numerous studies had focused on identifying the key microbial pathogens associated with AP and the revealed predominance of gram-negative anaerobes, for example, *Fusobacterium nucleatum, Treponema denticola, Tannerella forsythia*, and *Porphyromonas gingivalis*.[30–32] These bacteria yield lipopolysaccharide (LPS), playing key roles in eliciting the inflammatory responses in AP.[33,34] LPS binds to toll-like receptors 2 and 4 (TLR2 and TLR4), triggering signaling pathways that result in transcriptional activation of proinflammatory cytokines, for example, interleukin-1β (IL-1β), IL-6, IL-8, and tumor necrosis factor-α (TNF-α),[35,36] which in turn drive CD4$^+$ T-cell differentiation and recruitment of inflammatory cells to the site of pathogenesis.[37]

Periapical bone resorption in AP is tightly regulated by osteoclastogenesis through receptor activator of nuclear factor kappa B (RANK) ligand and osteoprogerin (OPG).[38,39] Exposure of osteoblasts to LPS induces RANK ligand, IL-1, TNF-α, and prostaglandin $E_2$, all of which induce osteoclastogenesis.[40,41] RANK ligand presented by osteoblasts bind to RANK receptor on osteoclast precursors, resulting in osteoclast differentiation and bone resorption.[42,43] OPG may function as a decoy receptor by binding RANK ligand in place of RANK and prevent RANK-mediated osteoclastogenesis, thereby suppressing bone resorption.[44,45] In AP, bone loss is driven by the RANK mechanism, whereas OPG level is largely undetected in periapical tissue fluid.[39,46] Among periapical granuloma tissues collected from infected root apices, RANK ligand expression is significantly upregulated when compared with normal PDL tissues. These granulomatous tissues contain monocytes and dendritic cells producing a significant amount of RANK ligand.[47] In fact, based on periapical tissue fluid samples collected from infected root apices, periapical bone resorption signaling by RANK ligand precedes recruitment of inflammatory cells by proinflammatory cytokines.[39] Thus, RANK ligand plays an important role in mediating osteoclastogenesis and bone destruction during the early stage of AP.

Periapical granulomas contain elevated levels of inflammatory cytokines and chemokines that facilitate inflammatory cell infiltration, resulting in active periapical tissue destruction. Jakovljevic and colleagues[48] reported highly elevated levels of IL-1β, IL-6, and TNF-α in symptomatic AP, representing active disease state, compared with asymptomatic AP; the same study also found further elevated IL-1β in radicular cysts compared with granulomatous lesions. Large, symptomatic, and epithelialized lesions exhibit significantly high levels of IL-6 and granulocyte-macrophage colony-stimulating factor when compared with asymptomatic, nonepithelialized lesions.[49] Using a rat AP model, Cintra and colleagues[50] showed elevated IL-6, IL-17, IL-23, and TNF-α levels in periapical granulomas and blood serum. Likewise, a rat AP model revealed elevation of chemokines, monocyte chemotactic protein (MCP-1), and chemokine receptor type 2 (CCR2) in periapical lesions.[51] Exploration of human AP samples also indicated increased level of CXCL12/SDF-1 chemotactic factors, which facilitate recruitment of wide array of leukocytes during inflammation as well as cells expressing chemokine receptors, for example, CCR3, CCR5, CXCR3.[52,53] These studies demonstrate the complexity of effector molecule network during the initiation and progression of AP.

Immune activation is marked by differentiation of naïve CD4$^+$ T-helper (Th) cells into specialized lineages, which include proinflammatory Th1 cells expressing interferon-$\gamma$ and TNF-$\alpha$ or immunomodulatory Th2 cells expressing IL-4, IL-5, and IL-13.[54] Naïve Th cells can also differentiate into Th17 or Treg cells through discrete action of specific cytokines, such as transforming growth factor-$\beta$ (TGF-$\beta$) and IL-6 or IL-2, respectively.[54] CD4$^+$ Th lineage is determined in part through expression of specific transcription regulators, for example, T-bet (Th1), GATA3 (Th2), FoxP3 (Treg), and ROR$\gamma$P (Th17), some of which are under the regulation of epigenetic modulators as discussed later in this article. To assess differential levels of Th subtypes in AP, periapical cysts and granulomatous lesions were assayed for the levels of Th markers, including T-bet, FoxP3, IL-4, IL-10, and TGF-$\beta$.[55] This study found predominance of Th1 response in periapical granulomas consistent with proinflammatory and osteoclastic activities, whereas Treg markers were also induced to balance the level of inflammation.

Following cytokine release, intracellular events downstream of cytokine receptor signaling led to the inflammatory effects through target gene activation. One example of intracellular cytokine signaling involves activation of the Janus kinase/signal transducers and activators of transcription (JAK/STAT) pathway. JAK responds to the number of inflammatory cytokines that bind to cognate cytokine receptors, which then leads to recruitment of STAT to the receptor for phosphorylation by JAK and nuclear translocation to drive the target gene expression.[56] Activated nuclear STAT molecules then transcriptionally regulate diverse array of cytokines and inflammatory modulators. One of the targets of STAT transcription factors includes suppressors of cytokine signaling (SOCS), which inhibit the JAK/STAT signaling and suppress osteoclast activation and bone destruction.[57,58] For instance, expression of SOCS1 and SOCS3 are induced by activated nuclear STAT, and these proteins in turn inhibit the kinase activity of JAK, thereby providing a negative feedback mechanism to suppress JAK/STAT signaling.[59] Pathogenesis of AP is tightly regulated through both proinflammatory and immunomodulatory cytokines. AP lesions presenting with periapical granulomas exhibit elevated TNF-$\alpha$ and RANKL for osteoclast differentiation[60] as well as elevated level of IL-10, an anti-inflammatory cytokine that inhibits osteoclastogenesis.[61,62] Furthermore, an earlier study reported elevated levels of SOCS1-3 and IL-10 in periapical granulomas, suggesting the role of immune suppressive factors that control the level of inflammatory tissue responses during AP.[60] Disease mechanism of AP with interplay between oral infection, cytokines, and immune cells is summarized in **Fig. 1**.

Although oral bacteria are the primary cause of AP, other factors also play an important role in exacerbation of the disease. Several studies demonstrate the association between smoking and increased incidence of AP.[63,64] Type 2 diabetes mellitus and poor glycemic control has also been identified as a risk factor, being associated with increased incidence of AP.[65,66] Beyond smoking and diabetes, recent evidence points to genetic predisposition to development of and severity of AP. Morsani and colleagues[67] demonstrated that IL-1$\beta$ gene polymorphisms, specifically allele 2 of IL-1$\beta$, result in a 4-fold increase in production of IL-1$\beta$ and increased susceptibility to AP. In addition to IL-1$\beta$, gene polymorphisms in IL-6 and TNF-$\alpha$ have also been associated with increased incidence of symptomatic dental abscesses.[68] Polymorphisms in matrix metalloproteinases (MMP2 and MMP3), which play an important role in bone resorption and periapical tissue destruction, have also been associated with increased incidence of periapical lesion formation.[69] Thus, AP is clearly a multifactorial disease that is exacerbated by smoking and certain systemic diseases and has a clear genetic predisposition.

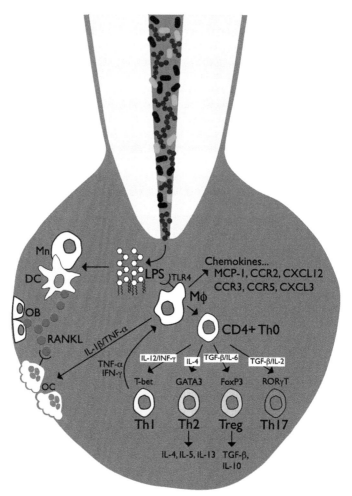

**Fig. 1.** Cellular and molecular constituents of AP. Root canal infection with microorganisms releases the inflammatory mediators, for example, LPS, which activates the inflammatory signaling in macrophages (MΦ), dendritic cells (DC), and monocytes (Mn). These reactions elicit proinflammatory cascades that increase secretion of RANKL from osteoblasts (OB) and DC, which promote osteoclast (OC) maturation through RANK surface receptor, resulting in bone resorption. Also, inflammatory signaling in AP is fueled by predominance of Th1 cells, which differentiate from CD4⁺ naïve Th (Th0) cells through Th1 transcription factor T-bet, whereas immunomodulatory Treg differentiation is also induced by FoxP3.

## EPIGENETIC REGULATION OF GENE EXPRESSION

Earlier studies on the pathogenesis of AP have thus far focused on the impact of the effector molecules, for example, TNF-α, IL-1β, RANKL, MCP-1, and other relevant cytokines, on the inflammatory bone resorption at periapex in a diseased tooth. However, the mechanisms that regulate the expression of these effector molecules are largely unknown and will be subject of investigation in the future. There has been growing interest in the role of epigenetics on gene regulation, in part due to the discovery of multiple epigenetic regulators, for example, histone Lys-specific demethylases (KDMs) and histone Lys methyltransferases (KMTs). Epigenetics had long been thought to represent heritable, permanent alteration in gene state, for example, X chromosome inactivation.[70] However, earlier studies demonstrate that epigenetic regulation of gene expression is versatile and dynamic.[29] In recent years, several KDMs were discovered to possess regulator roles in inflammation and immune signaling, and these epigenetic regulators are the subject of this article, as they may relate to periradicular pathoses.

"Epigenetics" refers to a mode of regulation that does not depend on the sequence of DNA base-pairs but on the secondary structure of DNA determined by histone modifications, for example, methylation, acetylation, or ubiquitination. DNA molecules generally wrap around histone octamers made up of 4 histone types, including H2A, H2B, H3, and H4, together forming DNA-histone complex called nucleosomes. By altering the posttranslational modification of histone tails of each nucleosome, the regional structure of chromatin may change; in a relaxed state, regulatory proteins, for example, transcription factors, may have access to the DNA for the initiation of transcription, while condensed chromosome would inactivate the gene expression.

KMTs generally bind to the promoter regions of target genes and add methyl-group onto specific Lys residues of H3 or H4, whereas KDMs remove the methyl-group from the Lys residues, which then allows subsequent biochemical events leading to recruitment of other regulatory factors to the nucleosome and altered gene expression. So far, there are more than 30 KDMs and equally diverse members of the KMT family of protein, and these KDM/KMTs exhibit their enzyme activities with specific histone Lys substrates as summarized in **Table 1**. Because a Lys residue has 3 available electronic valencies at the $\varepsilon$ amino group ($-NH_3^+$), it may be mono-, di-, or trimethylated by distinct KMTs for 1, 2, or 3 methyl-groups, respectively; also, specific KDMs will remove the methyl-group from the $\varepsilon$ amino group in a valency-specific manner. For instance, KDM6B, also known as Jmjd3, is a specific KDM for trimethylated Lys 27 (K27) on H3 (H3K27Me3), which is generally associated with inactive gene promoter.[71] By removing a methyl-group from H3K27Me3, Jmjd3 triggers the gene expression. The dynamics of this epigenetic regulation is best exemplified in the control of *INK4A* gene, which plays a pivotal role in cellular aging. *INK4A* encodes for p16[INK4A], a cyclin-dependent kinase inhibitor that allows for activation of retinoblastoma (Rb) during aging and causes cell cycle arrest.[72] The importance of p16[INK4A] for cellular aging has been demonstrated in replication-induced aging as well as stress- and oncogene-induced cellular aging.[73] In younger cells, *INK4A* gene remains silent through the action of *enhancer of zeste homologue 2* (EZH2) possessing methyltransferase activity specific for H3K27Me2 and other epigenetic regulators, including Bmi-1.[74] These proteins belong to the Polycomb-group (PcG) family genes, which were originally discovered in *Drosophila* as group of transcriptional repressors for homeotic genes; the name "Polycomb" came from the mutant phenotype on sex combs of fruit fly.[75] These PcG proteins play major roles in suppressing *INK4A*, thereby allowing continued cell proliferation due to absence of p16[INK4A] expression and consequent activation of Rb. During cellular aging, the level of Jmjd3 is elevated and is recruited to the promoter regions of *INK4A* to demethylate H3K27Me3 and enhance the expression of p16[INK4A], which then causes cell proliferation arrest and triggers senescence.[71] Therefore, the PcG and Jmjd3 proteins have antagonistic roles in target gene regulation through epigenetic mechanisms centered on the methylation state of H3K27. Interestingly, Jmjd3 is

**Table 1**
**Summary of Lys-specific demethylases/Lys-specific methyltransferases and their enzyme activities with specific histone Lys substrates**

| KDMs | KMTs | Histone Target | Effect on Transcription | KDM Function |
|---|---|---|---|---|
| KDM1A/LSD1 | SETD1A SET7 | H3K4Me2 | Repression | • Promotes DNA damage response[92] |
| | SUVR5 G9A | H3K9Me2 | Activation | • Regulates VEGF-A expression in prostate cancer[93] |
| | SET8 SUV420H1 | H4K20Me1/2 | Activation | • Activates Wnt/β-catenin signaling in colorectal tumors[94]<br>• Potent drug target against AML and many sarcomas[95,96] |
| KDM1B/LSD2 | SETD1A SET7 | H3K4Me2 | Repression | • Regulates DNA methylation, elevated in breast cancer[97] |
| KDM2A/FBXL11/ JHDM1A | SET2 | H3K36Me2 | Activation | • Promotes lung tumorigenesis via ERK1/2 signaling[98] |
| KDM2B/FBXL10/ JHDM1B | SETD1A SET7 | H3K4Me3 | Repression | • Regulates cell cycle progression and senescence[99] |
| | SET2 | H3K36Me2 | Activation | • Prevents adipogenic conversion of pluripotent cells[100]<br>• Promotes AML and pancreatic cancer[101,102] |
| KDM3A/JMJD1A/ JHDM2A KDM3B/JMJD1B/ JHDM2B KDM3C/JMJD1C/ JHDM2C | SUVR5 G9A | H3K9Me2 | Activation | • Regulates embryonic stem cell differentiation[103]<br>• Regulates spermatogenesis & reproductive function[104,105] |
| KDM4A/JMJD2A/ JHDM3A KDM4B/JMJD2B KDM4C/JMJD2C/ JHDM3C | SUV39H SETDB1 | H3K9Me3 | Activation | • Inhibits senescence; overexpressed in lung cancer[106] |
| | SET2 | H3K36Me3 | Activation | • Promote self-renewal of embryonic stem cells[103,107]<br>• Regulates osteogenic differentiation of mesenchymal stem cells[108] |
| KDM4D/JMJD2D | SUV39H SETDB1 | H3K9Me3 | Activation | • Promotes DNA damage response and DSB repair[109]<br>• Regulates spermatogenesis[110] |
| KDM5A/JARID1A KDM5B/JARID1B KDM5C/JARID1C KDM5D/JARID1D | SETD1A SET7 | H3K4Me3 | Repression | • Required for natural killer cell activation[111]<br>• Promotes carcinogenesis through E2F/Rb pathway[112]<br>• Mutation leads to intellectual disability[113] |
| KDM6A/UTX KDM6B/JMJD3 KDM6C/UTY | EZH1 EZH2 | H3K27Me3 | Activation | • Regulates mesenchymal stem cell differentiation[108,114]<br>• Promotes cell proliferation arrest & senescence[71]<br>• Regulates inflammatory signaling & T-cell differentiation[78,79] |

(continued on next page)

| | | Histone | Effect on | |
|---|---|---|---|---|
| KDMs | KMTs | Target | Transcription | KDM Function |
| KDM7A/JHDM1D | SUVR5 G9A | H3K9Me2 | Activation | • Regulates neural differentiation[115] |
| | EZH1 EZH2 | H3K27Me3 | Activation | • Prevents tumor growth by suppressing angiogenesis[116] |
| KDM7B/PHF8 | SUVR5 G9A | H3K9Me2 | Activation | • Regulates rRNA transcription and synthesis[117] |
| | SET8 SUV420H1 | H4K20Me1/2 | Activation | • Critical for neuronal development[118] |
| KDM7C/PHF2 | SMYD5 SUV420H2 | H4K20Me3 | Activation | • Tumor suppressor, downre-gulated in gastrointestinal cancer[119]  • Activates TLR4-specific inflammatory genes[120] |
| KDM8/JMJD5 | SET2 | H3K36Me2 | Activation | • Regulates cancer cell proliferation[121] |

**Table 1**
*(continued)*

one of the few KDMs associated with inflammatory signaling, and the opposing roles of PcG and Jmjd3 are also evident in this process.

## ROLE OF LYS-SPECIFIC METHYLTRANSFERASE AND LYS-SPECIFIC DEMETHYLASES IN INFLAMMATORY SIGNALING

A couple of years before the discovery of KDMs that can function as epigenetic modulators of dynamic gene expression regulation, Saccani and Natoli[29] reported alteration of H3K9 methylation status on promoter regions of select genes involved in inflammatory signaling, for example, macrophage-derived chemokine (MDC) and EBV-induced molecule 1 ligand chemokine (ELC), in dendritic cells exposed to LPS. Dimethylated H3K9 (H3K9Me2) is generally associated with inactive promoters. Thus, demethylation of H3K9Me2 would result in gene activation, which is precisely what the authors reported in the dendritic cells exposed to LPS. H3K9Me2 demethylation was linked with recruitment of RNA polymerase II (Pol II) to the promoter regions, allowing for the expression of MDC and ELC. Subsequently, Lys-specific histone demethylase (LSD1) was discovered as the first KDM that carried out histone demethylation as a means of dynamic gene regulation,[76] and KDM family members have been ascribed to regulatory roles in diverse biological processes, including cell cycle control, carcinogenesis, development, and inflammation.[77]

The first evidence linking KDMs to inflammation was found by screening for the KDMs that were induced in Raw264.7 cells exposed to LPS; within 2 hours of exposure, Jmjd3 was strongly induced, allowing for demethylation of H3K27Me3.[28] It was also found that Jmjd3 induction during inflammation was dependent on NF-κB activity, the master regulator of inflammation signaling, as evinced by the lack of Jmjd3 induction in the presence of IκBα (NF-κB repressor) or deletion of IKKγ in cells exposed to LPS.[78] Global readout of protein-DNA interactions by chromatin immunoprecipitation sequencing revealed recruitment of Jmjd3 to the transcription start sites of immune regulatory genes and inflammatory mediators, and Jmjd3 binding to the promoters coincided with Pol II recruitment.[78] Furthermore, in a recent study on the effects of Jmjd3 on naïve CD4$^+$ T-cell differentiation, Jmjd3 knockout led to preferential differentiation to Th2 and Treg subtypes, whereas Th1 and Th17 lineages were suppressed.[79] Given the fact that Th1 and Th17 CD4$^+$ lineages promote the proinflammatory responses whereas Th2 and Treg differentiation assume the immunomodulatory functions,[80] the above study further supports the proinflammatory role of Jmjd3 through altering the lineage differentiation of naïve CD4$^+$ T cells. The underlying mechanism by which Jmjd3 affects CD4$^+$ T-cell differentiation involves its roles in transcription regulation. For instance, T-bet is a transcription regulator absolutely required for Th1 lineage differentiation of naïve CD4$^+$ T cells.[81] In Th2 state, promoter regions of *Infg* gene coding for INF-$\gamma$, a pro-inflammatory cytokine, is enriched with the repressive histone mark H3K27Me3, suppressing the gene expression.[82] A subsequent study reported that T-bet recruits Jmjd3 to the promoter regions of *Infg* for epigenetic chromatin remodeling in Th1 cells to allow for gene expression.[83] Hence, Jmjd3 offers the first example by which KDM modulates inflammatory signaling through epigenetic mechanisms.

Because histone demethylation is a dynamic process, KDMs' activity is balanced by counteracting methyltransferase activities of KMTs. As discussed earlier in this article, Lys methylation of H3K27 is carried out by EZH2, which functions in combination with other protein subunits, for example, EED and Suz12, that make up the Polycomb Repressive Complex (PRC) 2.[84] PRC2 maintains the condensed chromatin state through H3K27Me3 and recruitment of PRC1 complex proteins, including Cbx, Bmi-1, and RING1B, which display E3 ubiqituin ligase activity on Lys 119 of H2A.[85] These protein complexes in PRC1 and PRC2 function in tandem to cause chromatin condensation and gene suppression, primarily through limiting access of transcriptional machinery to the promoter DNA sequences. In addition, an earlier study discovered that H2AK119 is mono-ubiquitinated by 2A-HUB, which is distinct from PRC1 but also demonstrates E3 ubiquitin ligase activity.[86] Through RNA profiling, this study showed that 2A-HUB is required for silencing of diverse genes, including several chemokines, for example, Cxcl/MIP2, Ccl5/Rantes, and Cxcl10/IP-10. Promoter analyses revealed direct binding of 2A-HUB at the chemokine promoters and enrichment of ubiquitinated H2AK119, which then interfered with transcription elongation by RNA Pol II. These findings suggest direct involvement of polycomb proteins in inflammatory signaling through epigenetic gene regulation. **Fig. 2** summarizes the competing actions of polycomb proteins and Jmjd3 for inflammatory gene expression.[87] Therefore, it is plausible to modulate the level of inflammatory responses, including those of periapical and periodontal diseases, by altering the balance between KDMs and KMTs on the promoter regions of inflammatory genes.

## EMERGING THERAPEUTICS FOR APICAL PERIODONTITIS

As discussed earlier in this article, current treatment modalities of RCT is highly efficacious with success rates exceeding 90%,[1–4] although cross-sectional studies still attest to relatively high prevalence of AP.[5] In recent years, a new approach in endodontic therapies involving pulp regeneration has gained great interest from both basic and clinical endodontic sciences because such innovative treatment approach may further enhance the outcomes. Root canal obturation using gutta percha and the sealer may no longer be the standard treatment protocol, given predictable outcome with revascularization. Resolution of AP and control of periapical inflammation would be the primary goal of revascularization. To that end, continued effort in developing effective anti-inflammatory therapeutics for periapex is fully justified.

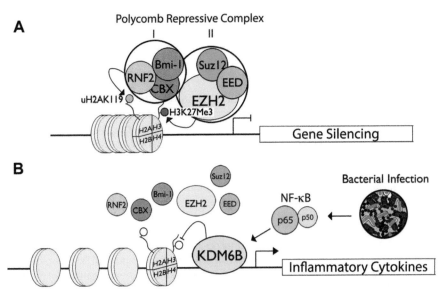

**Fig. 2.** Epigenetic role of KDM/KMTs during inflammation. (*A*) PRC I and II functions in tandem to maintain silencing of the genes, including those involved in inflammatory signaling. PRC II subunit EZH2 demonstrates KMT activity specific for H3K27Me3, which then is recognized by CBX of PRC I, leading to ubiquitination of H2AK119. Monoubiquitinated H2AK119 (uH2AK119) inhibits elongation of RNA Pol II and gene silencing.[86] (*B*) Upon bacterial infection, activation of NF-κB enhances the level of Jmjd3, a KDM specific for H3K27Me3, which is recruited to cytokine gene promoters. Demethylation of H3K27Me3 by Jmjd3 abrogates the PRC gene silencing activity, allowing for the expression of cytokine genes.

Because epigenetic regulation is positioned highly upstream in gene regulatory network, epigenetic modulators, for example, KMTs and KDMs, may affect diverse target genes and be an effective target for therapeutic drugs. For this reason, there has been growing interest in developing KDM inhibitors. For instance, vast majority of KDMs, those that contain peptide domain called Jumanji C (JmjC), require an enzyme cofactor α-ketoglutarate; these KDMs are effectively targeted by small compound 5-carboxyl-8-hydroxyquinoline.[88] Furthermore, a small molecule inhibitor for specific KDM has been developed based on 3-dimensional protein structure. Kruidenier and colleagues[89] reported GSK-J1/J4, which can selectively inhibit H3K27Me3 demethylases, including Jmjd3 and UTX. Subsequently, GSK-J4, the lipid soluble form of GSK-J1, has been used in other disease models in which Jmjd3 and/or UTX may have regulatory effects. Pediatric brainstem glioma is linked to mutations in Lys 27 of histone H3.3, causing shift in H3K27 methylation regulation by PcG proteins and Jmjd3.[90] Inhibition of Jmjd3 demethylase activity in pediatric glioma cells named K27M demonstrated antitumor activity in xenograft model,[91] demonstrating pharmacologic effects of KDM inhibitors in human diseases. As discussed earlier in this article, Jmjd3 has profound regulatory effects in proinflammatory cytokine gene expression induced by LPS exposure in macrophages and Th1 lineage differentiation of naïve CD4$^+$ T cells.[78,79] Therefore, targeting Jmjd3 would yield anti-inflammatory effects. In fact, the study by Kruidenier and colleagues[89] demonstrated marked reduction of TNF-α expression in human primary macrophages by GSK-J4 when exposed to LPS through H3K27Me3 demethylation and loss of RNA Pol II binding. These findings raise a possibility that KDMs may be a therapeutic target to control the inflammation through mechanism that is vastly different from existing anti-inflammatory pathways.

## SUMMARY

AP is the disease entity in clinical endodontics and has been the subject of intense investigation in terms of microbial cause, molecular mechanisms, and treatment modalities. Although conventional endodontic therapies are effective in resolving AP, persistence of the disease and emergence of pulp regeneration as new endodontic treatment call for further understanding of AP as the endodontic disease entity. Earlier studies focused on the effector molecules, for example, inflammatory cytokines and mediators, as well as the cellular elements, for example, macrophages, lymphocytes, and osteoclasts, of AP to delineate the mechanisms underlying AP. These earlier research efforts were fueled by the availability of the murine pulp exposure models with specific gene knockouts. However, the role of regulatory molecules in AP, for example, transcription factors and signaling molecules, are not well understood. Recent findings that illustrate the involvement of KDMs and KMTs in epigenetic gene regulation in diverse biological processes allow the further investigation the regulatory molecules of AP. In particular, Jmjd3 with demethylase activity for H3K27Me3 has been identified as a regulator of inflammatory signaling, although no studies have yet uncovered its role in AP. Future research endeavors dealing with these regulatory molecules of AP may provide novel strategies to control the disease and further enhance the success of endodontic therapies.

## ACKNOWLEDGMENTS

This study was supported in part by grants from the American Association of Endodontists Foundation. M.K. Kang is supported by Jack Weichman Endowed Fund.

## REFERENCES

1. Strindberg L. The dependence of the results of pulp therapy on certain factors: an analytic study based on radiographic and clinical follow-up examinations. Acta Odontol Scand 1956;14(Suppl):1–175.
2. Farzaneh M, Abitbol S, Lawrence HP, et al. Treatment outcome in endodontics—the Toronto Study. Phase II: initial treatment. J Endod 2004;30(5):302–9.
3. Friedman S, Abitbol S, Lawrence HP. Treatment outcome in endodontics: the Toronto Study. Phase 1: initial treatment. J Endod 2003;29(12):787–93.
4. Marquis VL, Dao T, Farzaneh M, et al. Treatment outcome in endodontics: the Toronto Study. Phase III: initial treatment. J Endod 2006;32(4):299–306.
5. Huumonen S, Suominen AL, Vehkalahti MM. Prevalence of apical periodontitis in root filled teeth: findings from a nationwide survey in Finland. Int Endod J 2016. [Epub ahead of print].
6. Chala S, Abouqal R, Abdallaoui F. Prevalence of apical periodontitis and factors associated with the periradicular status. Acta Odontol Scand 2011;69(6):355–9.
7. Song M, Park M, Lee CY, et al. Periapical status related to the quality of coronal restorations and root fillings in a Korean population. J Endod 2014;40(2):182–6.
8. Ng YL, Mann V, Rahbaran S, et al. Outcome of primary root canal treatment: systematic review of the literature - part 1. Effects of study characteristics on probability of success. Int Endod J 2007;40(12):921–39.

9. Sjogren U, Hagglund B, Sundqvist G, et al. Factors affecting the long-term results of endodontic treatment. J Endod 1990;16(10):498–504.

10. Liang YH, Li G, Wesselink PR, et al. Endodontic outcome predictors identified with periapical radiographs and cone-beam computed tomography scans. J Endod 2011;37(3):326–31.

11. Cardoso FG, Ferreira NS, Martinho FC, et al. Correlation between volume of apical periodontitis determined by cone-beam computed tomography analysis and endotoxin levels found in primary root canal infection. J Endod 2015;41(7): 1015–9.

12. Mehrvarzfar P, Akhlagi NM, Khodaei F, et al. Evaluation of isthmus prevalence, location, and types in mesial roots of mandibular molars in the Iranian population. Dent Res J (Isfahan) 2014;11(2):251–6.

13. Tam A, Yu DC. Location of canal isthmus and accessory canals in the mesiobuccal root of maxillary first permanent molars. J Can Dent Assoc 2002;68(1):28–33.

14. Adcock JM, Sidow SJ, Looney SW, et al. Histologic evaluation of canal and isthmus debridement efficacies of two different irrigant delivery techniques in a closed system. J Endod 2011;37(4):544–8.

15. Nair PN. On the causes of persistent apical periodontitis: a review. Int Endod J 2006;39(4):249–81.

16. Ricucci D, Siqueira JF Jr, Lopes WS, et al. Extraradicular infection as the cause of persistent symptoms: a case series. J Endod 2015;41(2):265–73.

17. Khemaleelakul S, Baumgartner JC, Pruksakom S. Autoaggregation and coaggregation of bacteria associated with acute endodontic infections. J Endod 2006;32(4):312–8.

18. Harn WM, Chen YH, Yuan K, et al. Calculus-like deposit at apex of tooth with refractory apical periodontitis. Endod Dent Traumatol 1998;14(5):237–40.

19. Song M, Kim HC, Lee W, et al. Analysis of the cause of failure in nonsurgical endodontic treatment by microscopic inspection during endodontic microsurgery. J Endod 2011;37(11):1516–9.

20. An GK, Morse DE, Kunin M, et al. Association of radiographically diagnosed apical periodontitis and cardiovascular disease: a hospital records-based study. J Endod 2016;42(6):916–20.

21. Scannapieco FA. Periodontal inflammation: from gingivitis to systemic disease? Compend Contin Educ Dent 2004;25(7 Suppl 1):16–25.

22. Scannapieco FA, Genco RJ. Association of periodontal infections with atherosclerotic and pulmonary diseases. J Periodontal Res 1999;34(7):340–5.

23. Velsko IM, Chukkapalli SS, Rivera-Kweh MF, et al. Periodontal pathogens invade gingiva and aortic adventitia and elicit inflammasome activation in alphavbeta6 integrin-deficient mice. Infect Immun 2015;83(12):4582–93.

24. Kakehashi S, Stanley HR, Fitzgerald RJ. The effects of surgical exposures of dental pulps in germ-free and conventional laboratory rats. Oral Surg Oral Med Oral Pathol 1965;20:340–9.

25. Wang CY, Stashenko P. Kinetics of bone-resorbing activity in developing periapical lesions. J Dent Res 1991;70(10):1362–6.

26. Sasaki H, Hou L, Belani A, et al. IL-10, but not IL-4, suppresses infection-stimulated bone resorption in vivo. J Immunol 2000;165(7):3626–30.

27. Stashenko P, Teles R, D'Souza R. Periapical inflammatory responses and their modulation. Crit Rev Oral Biol Med 1998;9(4):498–521.

28. De Santa F, Totaro MG, Prosperini E, et al. The histone H3 lysine-27 demethylase Jmjd3 links inflammation to inhibition of polycomb-mediated gene silencing. Cell 2007;130(6):1083–94.

29. Saccani S, Natoli G. Dynamic changes in histone H3 Lys 9 methylation occurring at tightly regulated inducible inflammatory genes. Genes Dev 2002; 16(17):2219–24.

30. Yoshimura A, Hara Y, Kaneko T, et al. Secretion of IL-1 beta, TNF-alpha, IL-8 and IL-1ra by human polymorphonuclear leukocytes in response to lipopolysaccharides from periodontopathic bacteria. J Periodontal Res 1997;32(3):279–86.

31. Fujii R, Saito Y, Tokura Y, et al. Characterization of bacterial flora in persistent apical periodontitis lesions. Oral Microbiol Immunol 2009;24(6):502–5.

32. Buonavoglia A, Latronico F, Pirani C, et al. Symptomatic and asymptomatic apical periodontitis associated with red complex bacteria: clinical and microbiological evaluation. Odontology 2013;101(1):84–8.

33. Schonfeld SE, Greening AB, Glick DH, et al. Endotoxic activity in periapical lesions. Oral Surg Oral Med Oral Pathol 1982;53(1):82–7.

34. Yamasaki M, Nakane A, Kumazawa M, et al. Endotoxin and gram-negative bacteria in the rat periapical lesions. J Endod 1992;18(10):501–4.

35. Rossol M, Heine H, Meusch U, et al. LPS-induced cytokine production in human monocytes and macrophages. Crit Rev Immunol 2011;31(5):379–446.

36. He W, Qu T, Yu Q, et al. LPS induces IL-8 expression through TLR4, MyD88, NF-kappaB and MAPK pathways in human dental pulp stem cells. Int Endod J 2013;46(2):128–36.

37. McAleer JP, Zammit DJ, Lefrancois L, et al. The lipopolysaccharide adjuvant effect on T cells relies on nonoverlapping contributions from the MyD88 pathway and CD11c+ cells. J Immunol 2007;179(10):6524–35.

38. Ritchlin CT, Haas-Smith SA, Li P, et al. Mechanisms of TNF-alpha- and RANKL-mediated osteoclastogenesis and bone resorption in psoriatic arthritis. J Clin Invest 2003;111(6):821–31.

39. Rechenberg DK, Bostanci N, Zehnder M, et al. Periapical fluid RANKL and IL-8 are differentially regulated in pulpitis and apical periodontitis. Cytokine 2014; 69(1):116–9.

40. Zou W, Bar-Shavit Z. Dual modulation of osteoclast differentiation by lipopolysaccharide. J Bone Miner Res 2002;17(7):1211–8.

41. Suda K, Udagawa N, Sato N, et al. Suppression of osteoprotegerin expression by prostaglandin E2 is crucially involved in lipopolysaccharide-induced osteoclast formation. J Immunol 2004;172(4):2504–10.

42. Yasuda H, Shima N, Nakagawa N, et al. Osteoclast differentiation factor is a ligand for osteoprotegerin/osteoclastogenesis-inhibitory factor and is identical to TRANCE/RANKL. Proc Natl Acad Sci U S A 1998;95(7):3597–602.

43. Udagawa N, Takahashi N, Jimi E, et al. Osteoblasts/stromal cells stimulate osteoclast activation through expression of osteoclast differentiation factor/RANKL but not macrophage colony-stimulating factor: receptor activator of NF-kappa B ligand. Bone 1999;25(5):517–23.

44. Simonet WS, Lacey DL, Dunstan CR, et al. Osteoprotegerin: a novel secreted protein involved in the regulation of bone density. Cell 1997;89(2):309–19.

45. Hsu H, Lacey DL, Dunstan CR, et al. Tumor necrosis factor receptor family member RANK mediates osteoclast differentiation and activation induced by osteoprotegerin ligand. Proc Natl Acad Sci U S A 1999;96(7):3540–5.

46. Liu D, Xu JK, Figliomeni L, et al. Expression of RANKL and OPG mRNA in periodontal disease: possible involvement in bone destruction. Int J Mol Med 2003; 11(1):17–21.

47. Vernal R, Dezerega A, Dutzan N, et al. RANKL in human periapical granuloma: possible involvement in periapical bone destruction. Oral Dis 2006;12(3):283–9.

48. Jakovljevic A, Knezevic A, Karalic D, et al. Pro-inflammatory cytokine levels in human apical periodontitis: correlation with clinical and histological findings. Aust Endod J 2015;41(2):72–7.

49. Radics T, Kiss C, Tar I, et al. Interleukin-6 and granulocyte-macrophage colony-stimulating factor in apical periodontitis: correlation with clinical and histologic findings of the involved teeth. Oral Microbiol Immunol 2003;18(1):9–13.

50. Cintra LT, Samuel RO, Azuma MM, et al. Multiple apical periodontitis influences serum levels of cytokines and nitric oxide. J Endod 2016;42(5):747–51.

51. Liu L, Wang L, Wu Y, et al. The expression of MCP-1 and CCR2 in induced rats periapical lesions. Arch Oral Biol 2014;59(5):492–9.

52. Cavalla F, Reyes M, Vernal R, et al. High levels of CXC ligand 12/stromal cell-derived factor 1 in apical lesions of endodontic origin associated with mast cell infiltration. J Endod 2013;39(10):1234–9.

53. Kabashima H, Yoneda M, Nagata K, et al. The presence of chemokine receptor (CCR5, CXCR3, CCR3)-positive cells and chemokine (MCP1, MIP-1alpha, MIP-1beta, IP-10)-positive cells in human periapical granulomas. Cytokine 2001; 16(2):62–6.

54. Zhu J, Yamane H, Paul WE. Differentiation of effector CD4 T cell populations (*). Annu Rev Immunol 2010;28:445–89.

55. Fukada SY, Silva TA, Garlet GP, et al. Factors involved in the T helper type 1 and type 2 cell commitment and osteoclast regulation in inflammatory apical diseases. Oral Microbiol Immunol 2009;24(1):25–31.

56. Cai B, Cai JP, Luo YL, et al. The specific roles of JAK/STAT signaling pathway in sepsis. Inflammation 2015;38(4):1599–608.

57. Narazaki M, Fujimoto M, Matsumoto T, et al. Three distinct domains of SSI-1/SOCS-1/JAB protein are required for its suppression of interleukin 6 signaling. Proc Natl Acad Sci U S A 1998;95(22):13130–4.

58. Morita Y, Naka T, Kawazoe Y, et al. Signals transducers and activators of transcription (STAT)-induced STAT inhibitor-1 (SSI-1)/suppressor of cytokine signaling-1 (SOCS-1) suppresses tumor necrosis factor alpha-induced cell death in fibroblasts. Proc Natl Acad Sci U S A 2000;97(10):5405–10.

59. Croker BA, Kiu H, Nicholson SE. SOCS regulation of the JAK/STAT signalling pathway. Semin Cell Dev Biol 2008;19(4):414–22.

60. Menezes R, Garlet TP, Trombone AP, et al. The potential role of suppressors of cytokine signaling in the attenuation of inflammatory reaction and alveolar bone loss associated with apical periodontitis. J Endod 2008;34(12):1480–4.

61. Evans KE, Fox SW. Interleukin-10 inhibits osteoclastogenesis by reducing NFATc1 expression and preventing its translocation to the nucleus. BMC Cell Biol 2007;8:4.

62. Park-Min KH, Ji JD, Antoniv T, et al. IL-10 suppresses calcium-mediated costimulation of receptor activator NF-kappa B signaling during human osteoclast differentiation by inhibiting TREM-2 expression. J Immunol 2009;183(4): 2444–55.

63. Segura-Egea JJ, Jimenez-Pinzon A, Rios-Santos JV, et al. High prevalence of apical periodontitis amongst smokers in a sample of Spanish adults. Int Endod J 2008;41(4):310–6.

64. Persic Bukmir R, Jurcevic Grgic M, Brumini G, et al. Influence of tobacco smoking on dental periapical condition in a sample of croatian adults. Wien Klin Wochenschr 2016;128(7–8):260–5.

65. Segura-Egea JJ, Jimenez-Pinzon A, Rios-Santos JV, et al. High prevalence of apical periodontitis amongst type 2 diabetic patients. Int Endod J 2005;38(8):564–9.

66. Sanchez-Dominguez B, Lopez-Lopez J, Jane-Salas E, et al. Glycated hemoglobin levels and prevalence of apical periodontitis in type 2 diabetic patients. J Endod 2015;41(5):601–6.

67. Morsani JM, Aminoshariae A, Han YW, et al. Genetic predisposition to persistent apical periodontitis. J Endod 2011;37(4):455–9.

68. de Sa AR, Moreira PR, Xavier GM, et al. Association of CD14, IL1B, IL6, IL10 and TNFA functional gene polymorphisms with symptomatic dental abscesses. Int Endod J 2007;40(7):563–72.

69. Menezes-Silva R, Khaliq S, Deeley K, et al. Genetic susceptibility to periapical disease: conditional contribution of MMP2 and MMP3 genes to the development of periapical lesions and healing response. J Endod 2012;38(5):604–7.

70. Peters AH, Mermoud JE, O'Carroll D, et al. Histone H3 lysine 9 methylation is an epigenetic imprint of facultative heterochromatin. Nat Genet 2002;30(1):77–80.

71. Agger K, Cloos PA, Christensen J, et al. UTX and JMJD3 are histone H3K27 demethylases involved in HOX gene regulation and development. Nature 2007; 449(7163):731–4.

72. Loughran O, Malliri A, Owens D, et al. Association of CDKN2A/p16INK4A with human head and neck keratinocyte replicative senescence: relationship of dysfunction to immortality and neoplasia. Oncogene 1996;13(3):561–8.

73. Collins CJ, Sedivy JM. Involvement of the INK4a/Arf gene locus in senescence. Aging Cell 2003;2(3):145–50.

74. Jacobs JJ, Kieboom K, Marino S, et al. The oncogene and Polycomb-group gene bmi-1 regulates cell proliferation and senescence through the ink4a locus. Nature 1999;397(6715):164–8.

75. Simon J. Locking in stable states of gene expression: transcriptional control during Drosophila development. Curr Opin Cell Biol 1995;7(3):376–85.

76. Shi Y, Lan F, Matson C, et al. Histone demethylation mediated by the nuclear amine oxidase homolog LSD1. Cell 2004;119(7):941–53.

77. Accari SL, Fisher PR. Emerging roles of JmjC domain-containing proteins. Int Rev Cell Mol Biol 2015;319:165–220.

78. De Santa F, Narang V, Yap ZH, et al. Jmjd3 contributes to the control of gene expression in LPS-activated macrophages. EMBO J 2009;28(21):3341–52.

79. Li Q, Zou J, Wang M, et al. Critical role of histone demethylase Jmjd3 in the regulation of CD4+ T-cell differentiation. Nat Commun 2014;5:5780.

80. Kennedy R, Celis E. Multiple roles for CD4+ T cells in anti-tumor immune responses. Immunol Rev 2008;222:129–44.

81. Szabo SJ, Sullivan BM, Stemmann C, et al. Distinct effects of T-bet in TH1 lineage commitment and IFN-gamma production in CD4 and CD8 T cells. Science 2002;295(5553):338–42.

82. Schoenborn JR, Dorschner MO, Sekimata M, et al. Comprehensive epigenetic profiling identifies multiple distal regulatory elements directing transcription of the gene encoding interferon-gamma. Nat Immunol 2007;8(7):732–42.

83. Miller SA, Mohn SE, Weinmann AS. Jmjd3 and UTX play a demethylase-independent role in chromatin remodeling to regulate T-box family member-dependent gene expression. Mol Cell 2010;40(4):594–605.

84. Conway E, Healy E, Bracken AP. PRC2 mediated H3K27 methylations in cellular identity and cancer. Curr Opin Cell Biol 2015;37:42–8.

85. Li Z, Cao R, Wang M, et al. Structure of a Bmi-1-Ring1B polycomb group ubiquitin ligase complex. J Biol Chem 2006;281(29):20643–9.

86. Zhou W, Zhu P, Wang J, et al. Histone H2A monoubiquitination represses transcription by inhibiting RNA polymerase II transcriptional elongation. Mol Cell 2008;29(1):69–80.

87. Kang MK, Mehrazarin S, Park NH, et al. Epigenetic gene regulation by histone demethylases: Emerging role in oncogenesis and inflammation. Oral Dis 2016. [Epub ahead of print].

88. Rotili D, Tomassi S, Conte M, et al. Pan-histone demethylase inhibitors simultaneously targeting Jumonji C and lysine-specific demethylases display high anticancer activities. J Med Chem 2014;57(1):42–55.

89. Kruidenier L, Chung CW, Cheng Z, et al. A selective jumonji H3K27 demethylase inhibitor modulates the proinflammatory macrophage response. Nature 2012; 488(7411):404–8.

90. Wu G, Broniscer A, McEachron TA, et al. Somatic histone H3 alterations in pediatric diffuse intrinsic pontine gliomas and non-brainstem glioblastomas. Nat Genet 2012;44(3):251–3.

91. Hashizume R, Andor N, Ihara Y, et al. Pharmacologic inhibition of histone demethylation as a therapy for pediatric brainstem glioma. Nat Med 2014;20(12): 1394–6.

92. Mosammaparast N, Kim H, Laurent B, et al. The histone demethylase LSD1/KDM1A promotes the DNA damage response. J Cell Biol 2013;203(3):457–70.

93. Kashyap V, Ahmad S, Nilsson EM, et al. The lysine specific demethylase-1 (LSD1/KDM1A) regulates VEGF-A expression in prostate cancer. Mol Oncol 2013;7(3):555–66.

94. Huang Z, Li S, Song W, et al. Lysine-specific demethylase 1 (LSD1/KDM1A) contributes to colorectal tumorigenesis via activation of the Wnt/beta-catenin pathway by down-regulating Dickkopf-1 (DKK1) [corrected]. PLoS One 2013; 8(7):e70077.

95. Fiskus W, Sharma S, Shah B, et al. Highly effective combination of LSD1 (KDM1A) antagonist and pan-histone deacetylase inhibitor against human AML cells. Leukemia 2014;28(11):2155–64.

96. Bennani-Baiti IM, Machado I, Llombart-Bosch A, et al. Lysine-specific demethylase 1 (LSD1/KDM1A/AOF2/BHC110) is expressed and is an epigenetic drug target in chondrosarcoma, Ewing's sarcoma, osteosarcoma, and rhabdomyosarcoma. Hum Pathol 2012;43(8):1300–7.

97. Katz TA, Vasilatos SN, Harrington E, et al. Inhibition of histone demethylase, LSD2 (KDM1B), attenuates DNA methylation and increases sensitivity to DNMT inhibitor-induced apoptosis in breast cancer cells. Breast Cancer Res Treat 2014;146(1):99–108.

98. Wagner KW, Alam H, Dhar SS, et al. KDM2A promotes lung tumorigenesis by epigenetically enhancing ERK1/2 signaling. J Clin Invest 2013;123(12): 5231–46.

99. Tzatsos A, Paskaleva P, Lymperi S, et al. Lysine-specific demethylase 2B (KDM2B)-let-7-enhancer of zester homolog 2 (EZH2) pathway regulates cell cycle progression and senescence in primary cells. J Biol Chem 2011;286(38): 33061–9.

100. Inagaki T, Iwasaki S, Matsumura Y, et al. The FBXL10/KDM2B scaffolding protein associates with novel polycomb repressive complex-1 to regulate adipogenesis. J Biol Chem 2015;290(7):4163–77.

101. He J, Nguyen AT, Zhang Y. KDM2b/JHDM1b, an H3K36me2-specific demethylase, is required for initiation and maintenance of acute myeloid leukemia. Blood 2011;117(14):3869–80.

102. Tzatsos A, Paskaleva P, Ferrari F, et al. KDM2B promotes pancreatic cancer via polycomb-dependent and -independent transcriptional programs. J Clin Invest 2013;123(2):727–39.

103. Loh YH, Zhang W, Chen X, et al. Jmjd1a and Jmjd2c histone H3 Lys 9 demethylases regulate self-renewal in embryonic stem cells. Genes Dev 2007;21(20): 2545–57.

104. Liu Z, Oyola MG, Zhou S, et al. Knockout of the histone demethylase Kdm3b decreases spermatogenesis and impairs male sexual behaviors. Int J Biol Sci 2015;11(12):1447–57.

105. Kuroki S, Akiyoshi M, Tokura M, et al. JMJD1C, a JmjC domain-containing protein, is required for long-term maintenance of male germ cells in mice. Biol Reprod 2013;89(4):93.

106. Mallette FA, Richard S. JMJD2A promotes cellular transformation by blocking cellular senescence through transcriptional repression of the tumor suppressor CHD5. Cell Rep 2012;2(5):1233–43.

107. Das PP, Shao Z, Beyaz S, et al. Distinct and combinatorial functions of Jmjd2b/ Kdm4b and Jmjd2c/Kdm4c in mouse embryonic stem cell identity. Mol Cell 2014;53(1):32–48.

108. Ye L, Fan Z, Yu B, et al. Histone demethylases KDM4B and KDM6B promotes osteogenic differentiation of human MSCs. Cell Stem Cell 2012;11(1):50–61.

109. Khoury-Haddad H, Nadar-Ponniah PT, Awwad S, et al. The emerging role of lysine demethylases in DNA damage response: dissecting the recruitment mode of KDM4D/JMJD2D to DNA damage sites. Cell Cycle 2015;14(7):950–8.

110. Iwamori N, Zhao M, Meistrich ML, et al. The testis-enriched histone demethylase, KDM4D, regulates methylation of histone H3 lysine 9 during spermatogenesis in the mouse but is dispensable for fertility. Biol Reprod 2011;84(6): 1225–34.

111. Zhao D, Zhang Q, Liu Y, et al. H3K4me3 demethylase Kdm5a is required for NK cell activation by associating with p50 to suppress SOCS1. Cell Rep 2016;15(2): 288–99.

112. Hayami S, Yoshimatsu M, Veerakumarasivam A, et al. Overexpression of the JmjC histone demethylase KDM5B in human carcinogenesis: involvement in the proliferation of cancer cells through the E2F/RB pathway. Mol Cancer 2010;9:59.

113. Santos-Reboucas CB, Fintelman-Rodrigues N, Jensen LR, et al. A novel nonsense mutation in KDM5C/JARID1C gene causing intellectual disability, short stature and speech delay. Neurosci Lett 2011;498(1):67–71.

114. Hemming S, Cakouros D, Isenmann S, et al. EZH2 and KDM6A act as an epigenetic switch to regulate mesenchymal stem cell lineage specification. Stem Cells 2014;32(3):802–15.

115. Huang C, Xiang Y, Wang Y, et al. Dual-specificity histone demethylase KIAA1718 (KDM7A) regulates neural differentiation through FGF4. Cell Res 2010;20(2):154–65.

116. Osawa T, Muramatsu M, Wang F, et al. Increased expression of histone demethylase JHDM1D under nutrient starvation suppresses tumor growth via downregulating angiogenesis. Proc Natl Acad Sci U S A 2011;108(51):20725–9.

117. Zhu Z, Wang Y, Li X, et al. PHF8 is a histone H3K9me2 demethylase regulating rRNA synthesis. Cell Res 2010;20(7):794–801.

118. Tsukada Y, Ishitani T, Nakayama KI. KDM7 is a dual demethylase for histone H3 Lys 9 and Lys 27 and functions in brain development. Genes Dev 2010;24(5): 432–7.

119. Lin CS, Lin YC, Adebayo BO, et al. Silencing JARID1B suppresses oncoge-
     nicity, stemness and increases radiation sensitivity in human oral carcinoma.
     Cancer Lett 2015;368(1):36–45.
120. Stender JD, Pascual G, Liu W, et al. Control of proinflammatory gene programs
     by regulated trimethylation and demethylation of histone H4K20. Mol Cell 2012;
     48(1):28–38.
121. Hsia DA, Tepper CG, Pochampalli MR, et al. KDM8, a H3K36me2 histone deme-
     thylase that acts in the cyclin A1 coding region to regulate cancer cell prolifer-
     ation. Proc Natl Acad Sci U S A 2010;107(21):9671–6.

# Contemporary Root Canal Preparation

## Innovations in Biomechanics

Ove Andreas Peters, DMD, MS, PhD[a],*,
Maria Guiomar de Azevedo Bahia, DDS, MS, PhD[b],
Erika Sales Joviano Pereira, DDS, MS, PhD[c]

### KEYWORDS

- Nickel titanium • Heat treatment • Glide path • Cyclic fatigue • Corrosion
- Outcomes

### KEY POINTS

- *Instrument design:* Current innovations include modifications in helical angle, taper, and longitudinal shape as well as kinematics. The intended improvements are prevention of threading in, less canal transportation, better canal wall preparation, and less fatigue accumulation.
- *Nickel titanium alloy:* There is a trend toward more martensitic (ie, more flexible alloy modifications), which is realized by varying heat treatment, specifically after grinding, so that the martensitic finish temperature for recent instruments is often greater than room temperature.
- *Testing methods:* In the absence of clinical evidence, most information discerning current root canal preparation instruments stems from various in vitro experiments, notably assessment of canal transportation, cyclic fatigue, and corrosion.

## INTRODUCTION

Engine-driven instrumentation is a mainstay in root canal therapy as it serves the goal of canal shaping while reducing the number of procedural errors.[1,2] The last decade in instrument development can be characterized by several key strategies:

- The use of more flexible alloys, which not only promise better canal negotiation but also extended fatigue life

Disclosures: Dr O.V. Peters serves as a consultant for Dentsply Tulsa Dental. Drs M.G. de Azevedo Bahia and E.S.J. Pereira deny any conflicts of interest.
[a] Department of Endodontics, University of the Pacific Arthur A. Dugoni School of Dentistry, 155 5th Street, San Francisco, CA, USA; [b] Department of Restorative Dentistry, Faculty of Dentistry, Universidade Federal de Minas Gerais, Belo Horizonte, Minas Gerais, Brazil; [c] Department of Dental Clinic, School of Dentistry, Federal University of Bahia, Salvador, Bahia, Brazil
* Corresponding author.
*E-mail address:* opeters@pacific.edu

Dent Clin N Am 61 (2017) 37–58
http://dx.doi.org/10.1016/j.cden.2016.08.002
0011-8532/17/© 2016 Elsevier Inc. All rights reserved.

- The introduction of reciprocation motion and the reduction of the number of instruments used per patient
- The design of instruments that physically touch and instrument a larger section of canal wall surface and at the same time decrease the need for coronal flaring

Although nickel-titanium (NiTi) alloy has been in use for root canal instrument manufacturing for more than 25 years, only relatively recently were manufacturing strategies diversified beyond microgrinding that was used for steel burs before (**Table 1**). Heat processing, either during forming the raw NiTi wire or after grinding, have established so-called controlled memory (CM) instruments with high martensitic crystal content may be dead soft and very flexible but only permit about 2% linear strain before nonrecoverable plastic deformation occurs.[3] With these differences in flexibility, distinct differences in fatigue resistance are observed: martensitic files have significantly extended life spans.[3]

Currently most practitioners use electric motors to power rotary instruments. These motors are also undergoing development. The ability to set a torque limit is common to most electric motors, but many models now allow reciprocating action.[4] Although this is not entirely new,[5] several NiTi instruments have been developed entirely for reciprocation motion with unequal angles of rotation. Reciprocation movement has been shown to be efficient and safe.[6] In particular, fatigue life span is extended with reciprocation.[7]

Irrigation effect of infected root canal systems can be facilitated by mechanical forces[8] and perhaps a scraping action of instruments along the canal walls,[9] several techniques were initiated in the last years, beginning with the so-called self-adjusting file[10] and most recently the irrigation enhancement device XP-Endo (FKG, La-Chaux-de-Fonds, Switzerland).

Root canal treatment is frequently discussed in terms of treating apical periodontitis; however, clinical functionality of a tooth for an extended period is an important

---

**Table 1**
**Summary of current innovative nickel-titanium root canal preparation instruments**

| Name | Manufacturer | Key Innovations | Production Process |
|------|-------------|-----------------|-------------------|
| HyFlex EDM | Coltene | Manufacturing process | Electrical discharge machining |
| ProTaper Gold | Dentsply Maillefer | Alloy | Grinding, heat treatment |
| ProTaper Next | Dentsply Maillefer | Off-center cross section | Grinding, heat treatment |
| SAF | ReDent Nova Henry Schein | Longitudinal design, concept, manufacturing | Laser cutting, heat treatment |
| TRUShape | Dentsply Tulsa Dental | Longitudinal design, concept | Grinding, heat treatment, form pressing |
| Vortex Blue | Dentsply Tulsa Dental | Alloy, variable helical angle | Grinding, heat treatment |
| WaveOne Gold | Dentsply Maillefer | Alloy, variations in rectangular cross sections | Grinding, heat treatment |
| XP-Endo | FKG/Brasseler | Manufacturing process, concept | Grinding, heat treatment, form pressing |

endodontic outcome.[11,12] A major factor for fracture susceptibility of endodontically treated teeth is the removal of bulk dentin during access[13,14]; therefore, canal preparation[15,16] strategies are being developed that retain more dentin,[17] specifically in the coronal root third.

The following explores recent innovations in instrument design, describes NiTi properties, and details relevant tests for current root canal preparation instruments.

## DESIGN ELEMENTS OF ROOT CANAL PREPARATION INSTRUMENTS

Historically, many root canal preparation instruments, such as K-files and later NiTi rotary instruments, followed certain design principles that relate to drills and reamers used for work in wood and metal. Design elements, such as the tip, flutes, and cross sections, are considered relevant for files and reamers used in rotary motion. These pertinent aspects and recent changes are briefly described later; for a more detailed review, the reader is referred to the literature.[18–20]

### Instrument Design: Tip, Cross section, Longitudinal Shape

In root canal preparation, an instrument tip has 2 main functions: to guide the file through the canal and to aid the file in penetrating deeper into the canal. An actively cutting tip[21,22] and file rigidity determine the propensity of a file to transport the canal; but as long as a flexible file with a noncutting tip the canal wall 360°, canal transportation is unlikely to occur.[23] Instrument tips have been previously described as cutting, noncutting, and partially cutting; however, current file tips are typically rounded and noncutting (**Fig. 1**). Comparatively little innovations in tip design have been noted in current instruments.

The cutting ability of a rotary instrument is determined to a large extent by its cross-sectional design. Seen in cross section (see **Fig. 1**), most current files have triangular or quadrangular cross sections, which result in negative rake angle. This angle is defined as the angle formed by the leading edge and the radius of the file through the point of contact with the radicular wall.

The cutting angle is considered a better indication of a file's cutting ability and is determined by measuring the angle formed by the leading edge of the file and a tangent to the radicular wall in the point of contact. Recent changes for

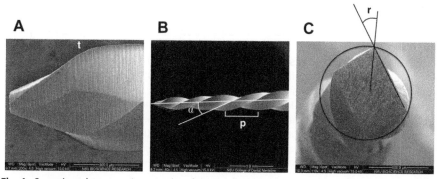

**Fig. 1.** Scanning electron micrographs of design features of a WaveOne Gold Primary instrument (Dentsply Maillefer). Magnifications are 200×, 40×, and 110×. (*A*) Tip design with smooth transition (*t*). (*B*) Lateral aspect with asymmetrical flute spacing, shown here are helical angle (*α*) and pitch (*p*). (*C*) Cross-sectional design with rectangular shape. Shown is rake angle (*r*). Note left-leaning spirals. (*Courtesy of* Sergio Kuttler, DDS, Fort Lauderdale, FL.)

cross-sectional design include variations in rectangular and parallelogram configurations and offset center points (see **Table 1**), which is intended to alternate radicular wall contact and possible reduce stress on the file; however, no data are currently available to validate these claims.

Seen in longitudinal view, typical NiTi rotaries show 2 to 4 flutes that have their leading edges spaced apart by a defined distance called pitch. The smaller the pitch or the shorter the distance between corresponding points, the more spirals are visible and the greater the helix angle will be (see **Fig. 1**). Similar to K-files, early rotary files, such as ProFile (Dentsply Tulsa, Tulsa, OK), had a constant pitch in the range of 1 mm. Current NiTi rotaries have a variable pitch, one that changes along the working surface. Pitch and helical angle are connected via the so-called *arctan* function shown in Equation 1:

$$\text{helical angle } \alpha = \arctan\frac{(\pi d)}{(sp)} \tag{1}$$

where $d$ is the local diameter of the instrument, $p$ is the pitch, and $s$ is the number of flutes.

The consequence is that instruments with a constant pitch will have a higher helical angle at the shank portion than at the tip. Changing the pitch had allowed the manufacture of instruments with defined helical angles (eg, RaCe, FKG; GT Rotary and GTX, Dentsply Tulsa Dental; and more recently, Vortex, Dentsply Tulsa Dental) (see also **Table 1**). The presumptive improvement of a helical angle that is higher at the tip and a lower at the shank includes less threading in; however, although some in vitro evidence exists in this regard,[24] a direct connection to clinical performance has yet to be established.

A longitudinal section through an instrument reveals the core, which can be tapered with similar deep fluting along the cutting portion. Alternatively, the core may be parallel with the consequence of a more flexible instrument toward the shank. Another design element visible in the longitudinal aspect is the file taper defined as a change in diameter per millimeter of working flutes. In other words, a 0.06-mm taper indicates that there is a linear change in diameter with an increment of 0.06 mm per millimeter. Current rotaries have either fixed or variable tapers; a variable taper permits the reduction of the maximum fluted diameter that can get to 1.2 mm and more in instruments with fixed tapers. So-called regressive tapers are evident in instruments, such as TRUShape (Dentsply Tulsa Dental), WaveOne Gold (Dentsply Maillefer), and V Taper (SS-White, Lakewood, NJ).

Changes in lateral design have given rise to specialized rotaries for glide path preparation that typically have a 0.02-mm taper and diameters equivalent to sizes No. 10 to No. 20, available from various manufacturers. The opposite of the spectrum are dedicated orifice shapers, also offered by several companies; these instruments have tip sizes of No. 20 and tapers of 0.08 mm.

The most radical changes for canal preparation instruments are perhaps embodied in the SAF (Redent-Nova, Ranaa, Israel) and TRUShape (**Figs. 2** and **3**); both are designed to adapt to nonround canal cross sections. Although the SAF is manufactured from a thin-walled and specifically cutout NiTi tube, TRUShape is press formed to create a sweeping S curve that is compressed as the instrument rotates in the canal.

In vitro evidence for both of these instruments, obtained with micro–computed tomography (micro-CT) suggests canal preparation with a high amount of prepared canal surface and minimal canal transportation.[25,26] The innovations described earlier depend largely on changes in NiTi alloy and manufacturing process, as detailed later.

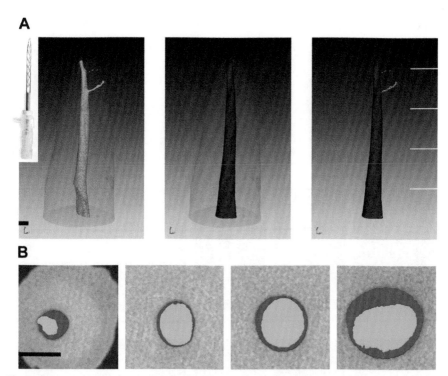

**Fig. 2.** Micro–computed tomography (MCT) to evaluate canal shaping with innovate instruments. Representative example of MCT data of maxillary anterior root canals prepared with the SAF (*inset, A*). Preparation time was 5 minutes; note almost complete preparation of canal surface. Black length bars are 1 mm; green and red areas are preoperative and postoperative cross sections, respectively. (*A*) Preoperative, postoperative, and superimposed MCT reconstructions (*from left to right*) demonstrating a patent lateral canal in the apical one-third of the root (volume, 0.033 mm³). (*B*) Cross sections at 1, 5, 9, and 13 mm coronal of the apex (*white lines* in *A*) detailing the amount of removed dentin along the canal perimeter. (*From* Peters OA, Boessler C, Paqué F. Root canal preparation with a novel nickel-titanium instrument evaluated with micro-computed tomography: canal surface preparation over time. J Endod 2010;36(6):1069; with permission.)

## NICKEL-TITANIUM ALLOYS: BASIC PROPERTIES AND IMPACT OF MANUFACTURING PROCESSES

In near equiatomic NiTi alloys, *shape memory effect* (SME) refers to the ability of certain materials to remember a shape, even after rather severe deformations: once deformed at low temperatures (in their martensitic phase), these materials will stay deformed until heated, whereupon they will spontaneously return to their original, predeformed shape. Superelasticity (SE) is associated with a large nonlinear recoverable strain on loading and unloading. Both SME and SE occur in association with the martensitic transformation from the parent phase (β) with a B2 structure to the phase with a monoclinic B19' structure.[27,28] The martensitic transformation is a so-called diffusionless phase transformation, in which atoms move cooperatively, often by a shearlike mechanism, without changing chemical composition of the matrix. The phenomena are sensitive to the fine structure of the parent β phase. Factors such as Ni content, aging, and thermomechanical treatment that affect this fine structure are

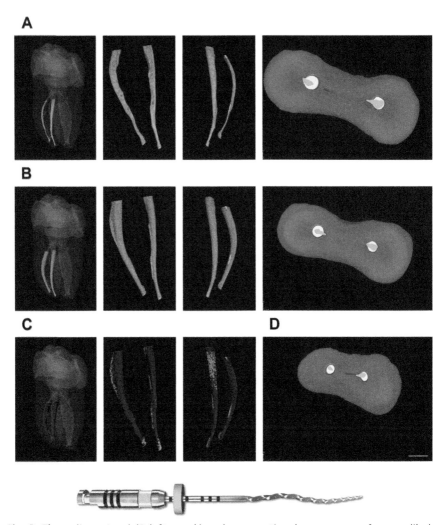

**Fig. 3.** Three-dimensional (*3 left panels*) and cross-sectional appearance of a mandibular molar, with the canal prepared with TRUShape shown on the right and Vortex shapes shown on the left. (*A*) Uninstrumented mesial canals; (*B*, *C*) the appearance after shaping to sizes No. 20 and 30, respectively. The panels in (*D*) show cross sections in the coronal, middle, and apical third, with the respective canal preparation steps indicated by yellow (size No. 20) and red (size No. 30). Scale bar = 1 mm. The insert at the bottom is the TRUShape rotary size No. 20 .06v. (*From* Peters OA, Arias A, Paqué F. A micro–computed tomographic assessment of root canal preparation with a novel instrument, TRUShape, in mesial roots of mandibular molars. J Endod 2015;41(9):1547; with permission.)

important for controlling the superelastic and memory behavior. Although fully annealed equiatomic NiTi alloys transform from the B2 parent phase to the monoclinic B19' phase, thermally cycled or thermomechanically treated NiTi alloys transform in 2 steps (ie, from the B2 to the R phase and then to the B19' phase). The B2-R transformation is also martensitic. The 2-step transformation occurs in Ni-rich NiTi alloys aged at an appropriate temperature and in ternary NiTi alloys.[27,29]

The physical properties of martensite and austenite are different; by the phase transformation, a variety of significant property changes occur. The abbreviations $M_s$, $M_f$, $A_s$ and $A_f$ refer to the temperature at which the transformation to martensite starts ($M_s$) and finishes ($M_f$) and the temperatures at which the reversion austenite ($A_s$) starts and finishes ($A_f$), respectively (**Fig. 4**). The SME occurs when a specimen is deformed at less than $M_f$ or at temperatures between $M_f$ and $A_s$, greater than at which the martensite becomes unstable, and regains its original shape, by reverse transformation, on heating to a temperature greater than $A_f$. In this process, the shape of the specimen does not change because the transformation occurs in a self-accommodation manner. Thus, if external stress is applied, the twin boundaries

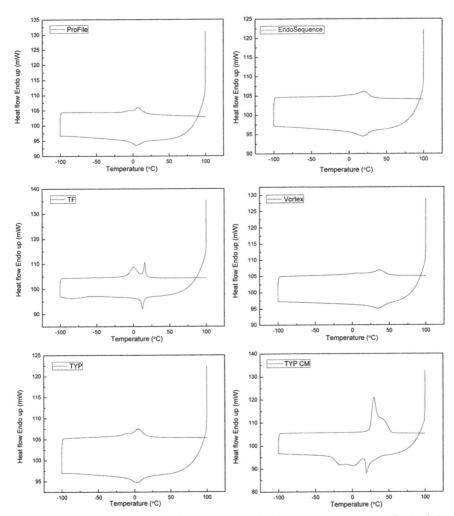

**Fig. 4.** Differential scanning calorimetry curves of the test specimens (ProFile, EndoSequence, Twisted File [TF], Vortex, Typhoon [TYP], and Typhoon CM [TYP CM]). Heating (*upper*) and cooling (*lower*) curves are shown. (*From* Shen Y, Zhou H, Zheng Y, et al. Metallurgical characterization of controlled memory wire nickel-titanium rotary instruments. J Endod 2011;37(11):1567; with permission.)

move so as to accommodate the applied stress; if the stress is high enough, it will become a single variant of martensite under stress, which is most favored by the applied stress. When the specimen is heated at greater than $A_f$, reverse transformation (RT) occurs; if the RT is crystallographically reversible, the original shape is regained. The deformation may be of any kind, such as tension, compression, or bending.[27,29]

One property that changes in a significant way is the yield strength. The martensitic structure can deform by moving boundaries of twins, which are quite mobile. Thus the yield strength of the martensite is extremely low compared with that of the austenite, which must deform by dislocation generation and movement. Only a certain amount of martensitic deformation can be accommodated by this twin movement process and once this is exceeded, the material will again deform elastically and eventually yield a second time by irreversible processes (dislocation movement).[29]

SE occurs by the stress-induced transformation on loading and the subsequent RT on unloading. Both SME and SE are closely related phenomena; the relation between the two is schematically shown in **Fig. 5**. SME at temperatures less than $A_s$, followed by heating greater than $A_f$, whereas SE occurs greater than $A_f$, whereby martensite is unstable in the absence of stress. In the temperature regimen between $A_s$ and $A_f$, both occur partially. In **Fig. 5**, a straight line with a positive slope represents the critical stress to induce martensite and the straight lines with negative slopes (A or B) represent the critical stress for slip. Because slip never recovers on heating or unloading, the stress must be below the line to realize SME and SE. It is clear that no SE is realized, if the critical stress is as low as the line B, because slip occurs before the onset of stress-induced martensite. Therefore, the essential conditions for the realization of SME and SE are the crystallographic reversibility of martensitic transformation and

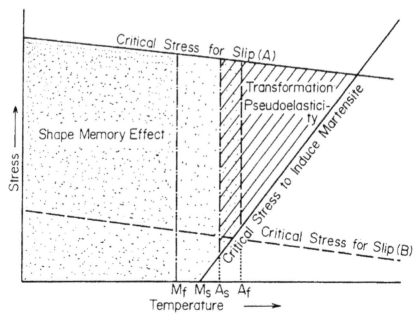

**Fig. 5.** The appearance of SME and superelasticity, which is termed *transformation pseudoelasticity* here, in temperature-stress space. (*From* Otsuka K, Ren X. Physical metallurgy of Ti–Ni-based shape memory alloys. Progress in Materials Science 2005;50(5):589; with permission.)

the avoidance of slip during deformation. It is expected that SME and SE characteristics may be improved by hardening of alloys for obtaining a higher critical stress for slip.[27]

There are 3 ways to increase the critical stress for slip:

1. Solution hardening
2. Precipitation hardening
3. Work hardening

After the discovery of the SME by William J. Buehler in 1963, the phase diagram of the NiTi alloys system was extensively reexamined because it is important for heat treatment of the alloys and improvement of the shape memory characteristics. Although in the equilibrium phase diagram of the NiTi system, the B2 phase region is very narrow (between 50.0 and 50.5 atomic % Ni) at temperatures less than 650°C. In these circumstances, NiTi alloys decompose on cooling slowly from a high temperature or on aging at temperature less than 700°C after quenching from high temperatures. The boundary on the Ni-rich side decreases greatly with decreasing temperature, and the solubility becomes negligible at about 500°C. It has been found that 3 phases $Ti_3Ni_4$, $Ti_2Ni_3$ (intermediate phases), and $TiNi_3$ (equilibrium phase) appear depending on annealing temperature and time. At lower aging temperature and shorter aging time. Precipitation of the $Ti_3Ni_4$ phase is very useful in adjusting transformation temperatures and in designing heat treatment because it strengthens the matrix B2 phase and, thus, improves the recoverability of the SME.[29,30]

### *Modification of Transformation Temperatures by Heat Treatment*

NiTi alloys with a small excess of Ni respond well to heat treatment at lower temperatures because coherent, submicroscopic $Ti_3Ni_4$ precipitates can form within the β-phase matrix.[31] Because the $Ti_3Ni_4$ precipitates contain more Ni than Ti, their formation decreases the amount of Ni in solid solution and increases the transformation temperatures, which are sensitive to the Ni content.[32] As shown before, transformation temperature determines at what temperature (range) the martensitic transformation can be observed. This point is very important for practical applications, and there are 2 ways of changing/controlling transformation temperature (ie, by composition and by annealing treatment). A useful possibility is to use the precipitation reaction of equiatomic alloys to finely adjust the composition of the NiTi matrix and, hence, give a precise control of transformation temperature. The principle is the (metastable) equilibrium between NiTi and $Ti_3Ni_4$ precipitates. Although $Ti_3Ni_4$ is considered as a metastable phase compared with the equilibrium $TiNi_3$ precipitate, it is quite stable at temperatures less than 600°C. Under normal annealing conditions only $Ti_3Ni_4$ is observed. As the $Ti_3Ni_4$ precipitates contain more Ni than Ti, their formation decreases the amount of Ni in solid solution and increases the transformation temperatures, which are sensitive to the Ni content.[29]

### *Metallurgical Characterization of Thermomechanically Treated Nickel-Titanium Instruments*

A series of studies[33–35] found that changes in the transformation behavior via heat treatment were effective in increasing the flexibility of NiTi endodontic instruments. Alapati and colleagues[36] indicated that heat treatments between 400°C and 600°C increased the $A_f$ temperature of NiTi files and heat treatment at 850°C caused a loss of SE behavior and recrystallization of the wrought microstructure. The value of the material's temperature in relation to test or clinical use temperatures is important to define the phases present in that condition. As mentioned earlier, NiTi alloys with a small excess of Ni respond well to heat treatment at lower temperatures because coherent, submicroscopic $Ti_3Ni_4$ precipitates can form within the β-phase matrix.[31] Because of their small size and coherence with the matrix, these precipitates increase the mechanical strength of austenite, helping to prevent plastic deformation on straining, and, thus, favoring the occurrence of stress-induced martensitic transformation that is paramount to the SE of the alloy.[32]

The results by differential scanning calorimetry (DSC) (see **Fig. 4**)[37] have shown that the NiTi instruments that were made using M-Wire (Sportswire LLC, Langley, OK, later marketed by Dentsply Tulsa Dental) and CM technologies exhibited $A_f$ temperatures between 33°C and 55°C. This finding indicates that a reasonable amount of martensite should be present in these instruments at the test temperature, whereas the NiTi instruments that were made from conventional NiTi exhibited $A_f$ temperatures of approximately room temperature. These data are consistent with previous studies,[38–40] which showed that instruments made from conventional NiTi alloys exhibit an austenitic phase at room temperature during clinical applications, whereas M-Wire and CM instruments, in addition to the austenite, also contained martensite B19′ and R phase.[3,41,42]

The realization that the mechanical properties of near equiatomic NiTi alloys are strongly influenced by the stress-induced phase transformation that takes place in this alloy and that the microstructural changes introduced by thermomechanical treatments can control this phase transformation constitutes the modern trend toward developing new rotary endodontic instruments with improved mechanical properties. There has been considerable improvement in file design, manufacturing methods and preparation techniques on rotary endodontic instruments made of NiTi alloys; however, intracanal fracture of instruments caused by flexural (cyclic) fatigue remains a primary concern in clinical practice, especially for canals with curvatures.[43] As mentioned before, mechanical performance of NiTi alloy is sensitive to its microstructures and associated thermomechanical history.[29] With the aim of improving the current NiTi alloy properties, a proprietary method of thermomechanical treatment of 508 Nitinol wire (Nitinol Devices & Components, Fremont, CA) was developed, now known as M-Wire. It includes some amount of both the R-phase and the B19′ martensitic phases,[44] while maintaining the alloy's superelasticity.[36,41,45,46] In such a thermomechanical procedure, the raw wire has undergone a processing method composed of thermomechanically treating under specific tensile stresses and temperatures. First of all, it is said that this treatment is to be performed on conventional nitinol wire after cold drawing in the martensitic phase to the finished diameter and annealed in the temperature interval 400°C to 475°C. The wire is then subjected to thermal cycling between a low-temperature bath (less than 10°C) and a high-temperature one (up to 180°C) 3 to 5 times under a strain in the superelastic regime.[47] Although the effect of this thermomechanical cycling is complex, it is known that thermal cycling under load has the potential to increase the starting temperature for the formation of B19′ martensite but has little effect on the R-phase starting temperature.[48] This could be the reason why both B19′ and the R phase coexist in M-Wire at room temperature and, thus, is compatible with the higher transformation temperatures found by DSC.

Alapati and colleagues[36] carried out the first metallurgical characterization of M-Wire, demonstrating that it had higher transformation temperatures compared with a conventionally treated NiTi wire used for the manufacture of NiTi instruments. These results were confirmed in a more recent study,[41] which showed that M-Wire had a lower apparent elastic modulus as well as smaller transformation stress and mechanical hysteresis. Some investigators found significantly higher resistance in the flexural fatigue (150%–400%) and improved flexibility of rotary instruments made of M-Wire compared with conventional NiTi.[38,46,49–51] It has been reported that NiTi instruments with higher transformation temperatures are more flexible[34,52] and that heat treating these instruments can increase the transformation temperatures[35] and improve this property.[35,53] However, the greater flexibility of instruments made with M-Wire should be attributed to their lower initial apparent elastic modulus, which can be associated with the stress-induced reorientation of the R-phase and B19′ martensite.[48] This material exhibits more efficient superelastic behavior with reduced generation and accumulation of lattice defects during each load-unload cycle,[41] increasing the fatigue resistance of these instruments.[38]

According to the literature[46,49–51,54] experimental and commercial instruments made with M-Wire exhibited better fatigue properties than instruments conventionally produced. As commented earlier, the superelastic plateau of the M-Wire specimen was achieved under a lower tensile stress.[41] Additionally, the stress at the plateau remained relatively constant until 6% elongation was attained (8 MPa), whereas this stress in conventional wire tended to increase in the same region (16 MPa).[41] This increase is the result of work hardening, which can take place in the superelastic region associated with a certain amount of plastic deformation.[29,30] Thus, more lattice defects were introduced in conventional NiTi than in M-Wire when the wires underwent the load/unload cycle. When this reasoning is applied to the rotary endodontic instruments made from these wires, it is easy to understand why those in which M-Wire was used presented higher fatigue resistance.[46,49–51,54] The reason is that the thermomechanical treatment applied to M-Wire led to a more efficient superelastic behavior with less generation and accumulation of lattice defects in each load-unload cycle.[41]

In 2008, a new manufacturing process was developed by SybronEndo (Orange, CA) to create a NiTi endodontic instrument marketed as Twisted-File (TF). According to the manufacturer, TF files were fabricated using a twisting method by transforming a raw NiTi wire in the austenite phase into the R phase through a thermal process. This proprietary technology was used to optimize the phase constituents and properties of TF files. Once the R phase is identified, wire in this state can be twisted. After additional thermal procedures to maintain its new shape, the instrument is converted back into the austenite phase, which is superelastic once stressed. It has been reported to have a higher flexibility and fatigue fracture resistance than ground files.[55–58] Another recent innovation is the use of spark erosion to manufacture HyFlex EDM (Coltene, Cuyahoga Falls, OH); according to the manufacturer this process uses electrical discharges of high energy to shape the file flutes rather than grinding or twisting processes. It seems from initial data for rotaries manufactured this way that mechanical properties, such as fatigue resistance and surface quality, are at least as good as with ground NiTi.[59]

As mentioned earlier, relative proportions and characteristics of the microstructural phases determine the mechanical behavior of NiTi alloys. Heat treatment is one of the most fundamental approaches toward adjusting transition temperatures of these alloys, with the objective of controlling the alloy microstructure and, thus, influencing its mechanical behavior.[3,60] Another example is CM technology in which endodontic instruments are subjected to a special thermal process after machining from conventional NiTi wire to increase their fatigue resistance.[39] However, despite the strong influence these parameters exert on the fatigue resistance of NiTi rotary files, information concerning the thermal treatment of raw materials and instruments currently remains limited because such heat treatments are generally proprietary and are not disclosed by manufacturers beyond published patents. CM technologies use special thermal processes to control the transition temperatures, making the instruments extremely flexible at room temperature because of the presence of martensite.[3,61] These production techniques are usually targeted toward increasing file flexibility and strength, which are thought to enhance the endodontic treatment efficiency and reduce the rate of iatrogenic errors. Thermomechanical treatment of NiTi alloy has a strong impact on its transformation behavior.[29] Instruments with CM showed a lower bending moment than the others probably because they are made of an alloy that features the R-phase and B19′ martensite; hence, there is a lower apparent modulus of elasticity at room temperature.[3,41,44,62] This finding means that at the beginning of the stress-strain curve of the material, the inclination of the curve is lower for CM NiTi compared with superelastic NiTi and the stress plateau is reached at a lower stress for the first alloy in which the phenomenon taking place is nothing but reorientation of previously existing martensite.[41,61]

It seems that a hybrid (austenite-plus-martensite) microstructure exhibiting a certain proportion of martensite, such as that observed in the M-Wire and CM files, is more likely to exhibit favorable fatigue resistance compared with a fully austenitic microstructure because of the significant number of interfaces present. These interfaces are known to cause the formation of complex arrays of secondary cracks, which can dissipate the energy required for crack propagation.[63] In addition, the presence of these martensitic structures has the potential of hardening the heat-treated alloys, as recently reported,[44,64] ruling out the possibility that the treatments involved in M-Wire and CM technologies may compromise the torsional resistance of endodontic instruments.

The fracture surfaces of fatigue-tested instruments observed by scanning electron microscopy exhibited the typical features of this fracture mode. The secondary electron images exemplify the larger areas of nucleation and slow crack propagation found in the CM instruments compared with the other instruments. Fatigue striations and secondary cracks were observed within the smooth regions of the fracture surface at a higher magnification, confirming that the instruments failed because of fatigue.[37,38,65,66]

Torsional strength is related to how much a file can twist before fracture and is desirable in the preparation of narrow and constricted canals because the file is subjected to high torsional loads. Studies analyzing the mechanical behavior of CM files showed that instruments that received specific heat treatments presented similar torsional resistance compared with instruments made of superelastic alloy, although they had significantly higher deformation before failure compared with conventional NiTi instruments.[37,62,66-70] One possible explanation for this could be that all instruments were deformed until the complete transformation to martensite took place; thus, failure occurred for all of them at the ultimate tensile strength of this phase.[44]

Some studies[62,71] showed that CM files exhibited a significantly higher angular deflection compared with M-Wire and conventional NiTi instruments. This feature may be associated with additional deformation provided by the reorientation of martensite in the first files. Furthermore, this characteristic can be understood as a higher safety factor if one decides to reuse rotary files because instruments showing more detectable distortion of the cutting spirals are more likely to be discarded before breakage.[62]

These current developments provide clinicians with an important understanding of the properties and differences of these materials so that they may take advantage of the latest technology.

## TESTING METHODS FOR CURRENT ROOT CANAL PREPARATION INSTRUMENTS

Because of their mechanical properties discussed earlier, rotary instruments made of NiTi alloys are commonly used clinically shaping of root canals that exhibit complex anatomies.[37] Despite the favorable properties of these alloys, a high risk of fracture continues to be a problem during endodontic therapy; metal fatigue represents a predominant reason for file separation.[72] Flexural fatigue fractures occur as a result of repeated compressive and tensile stresses that accumulate at the point of maximum flexure when instrument rotates within a curved canal.[43,73] Strain levels attained by rotary endodontic instruments during clinical use depend on the root canal geometry and the applied loads that are concentrated on the region of maximum curvature within the root canal, which can vary with the instrument diameter.[43,74] New rotary and reciprocating systems manufactured from NiTi alloy heat treated in a specific manner have a surface layer of titanium oxide (HyFlex, Vortex Blue, WaveOne Gold, TRUShape, see **Table 1**) and an increased fatigue resistance, besides greater flexibility than those made of conventional NiTi alloy. Thus, parameters such as cutting efficiency and the electrochemical potential in a corrosive environment become important as they address the following questions: To be more flexible, is their cutting power effective? Is the titanium oxide layer on its surface rendering these instruments more or less resistant to corrosion? Therefore, cutting efficiency, fatigue, and corrosion are parameters to be studied the new technologies in terms of NiTi endodontic instruments.

### Cutting Ability

Mechanical forces applied to NiTi instruments during endodontic canal preparation are complex and multiaxial,[24] which makes assessment of their cutting ability difficult. A direct comparison between instruments was performed with different testing devices using test blocks[24,75,76] or human dentin discs.[77]

Morgental and colleagues[78] evaluated the influence of rotational speed and number of uses on the cutting efficiency of 4 NiTi coronal flaring instruments made from different alloys. They found that HyFlex instruments made from CM alloy were the most cutting efficient instrument in lateral action. Peixoto and colleagues[79] described a device that measured torque and apical force of the file moved into the artificial canal under a constant insertion rate to assess cutting ability in axial motion. In their study, cross-sectional design, in particular for Mtwo 20/.06 (VDW, Munich, Germany) instruments with a 2-flute cross section, resulted in better cutting ability in comparison with ProTaper Universal F1 (Dentsply Tulsa Dental) and RaCe 20/.06 (FKG) instruments.

A recent study investigated the effect of repeated simulated clinical use and sterilization on cutting efficiency and flexibility of HyFlex CM rotary files. Cutting efficiency was determined by measuring the load required to maintain a constant feed rate, whereas instrumenting simulated canals and flexibility was determined by using a 3-point bending test. Repeated simulated clinical use and sterilization showed no effect on cutting efficiency through 1 use and no effect on flexibility through 2 uses.[80]

### Fatigue Testing

In the absence of establishes norms, studies evaluating flexural fatigue resistance of NiTi rotary files used testing setup, such as steel grooves, steel slopes, or 3-point steel pins, to guide the file into the desired curvature (**Fig. 6**)[37,46,57,67,81–83] and run

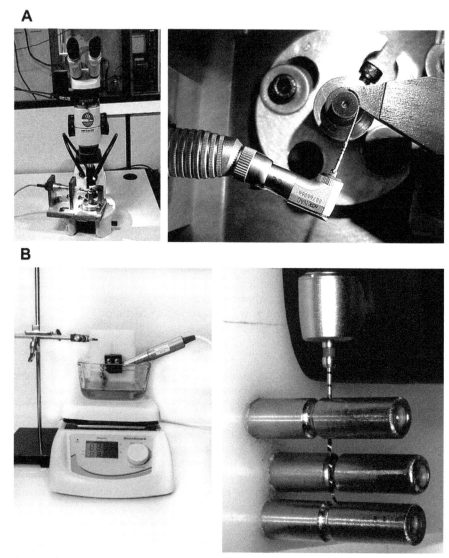

**Fig. 6.** Different approaches to fatigue testing to determine the numbers of cycles until failure. (*A*) Form block and rod assembly. (*B*) Steel peg assembly. Note higher magnification images that show the specific arrangements.

instruments at manufacturer recommended revolutions per minute until they break; the number of cycles until failure (NCF) is then calculated. However, radii and angles of curvature of the testing devices are often different, despite the fact that these two parameters have a significant effect on the fatigue resistance of rotary NiTi instruments.[43,73]

In fatigue analysis, instruments of similar geometric designs should be chosen for comparison. The instrument diameter at the point of the maximum canal curvature has been identified as the most important factor in the control of fatigue resistance of endodontic files.[43,44,74,84] The critical parameter is maximum tensile strain amplitude ($\epsilon_T$), which is determined using Equation 2:

$$\text{strain amplitude } \epsilon T = \frac{d}{(2r - d)} \tag{2}$$

where r is the canal radius measured at the outer canal wall and d is the local instrument diameter.

Johnson and colleagues[46] compared fatigue resistance of 508 Nitinol alloy and an experimental alloy that was later marketed as M-Wire NiTi. ProFile 25/.04 rotary instruments manufactured from M-Wire NiTi variant had up to 390% increased resistance to flexural fatigue compared with the same instrument design produced from stock 508.

A study by Braga and colleagues[37] considering a maximum tensile strain amplitude of about 5.3% to 5.5% in a curved artificial canal found increased fatigue resistance exhibited by the HyFlex and Typhoon (DS Dental, Johnson City, TN) files attributable to superior mechanical properties of CM wire used in both instruments.

Another study found that file manufacturing methods had an effect on fatigue resistance, specifically NiTi rotary files produced using a twisting process were superior to traditional NiTi instruments produced by grinding.[57]

Yet another recent fatigue study[67] used a model in which NiTi instruments were constrained to a curvature by 3 steel pins and run in a water bath at room temperature. Under those conditions, CM files had 7 times higher cycles to fatigue failure than files of the same design made from conventional NiTi alloy; no difference in torsional resistance was found.

Capar and colleagues[85] tested fatigue resistance of NiTi pathfinding instruments and found the following ranking (from highest to lowest NCF): HyFlex Glide Path File (Coltene), G-files (MicroMega), ProGlider, PathFile (both Dentsply Maillefer), and Scout Race (FKG).

Gao and colleagues[86] found for instruments with identical geometric design and different raw materials that heat treatment resulted in an titanium oxide layer with a Vickers hardness in the range of 620 to 970. They also determined that the heat-treated blue alloy was significantly more flexible and fatigue resistant, followed by M-Wire, superelastic wire, and stainless steel in a file of the same design.

Plotino and colleagues[81] confirmed these findings showing that Vortex Blue has superior flexural fatigue resistance when compared with the same sizes of ProFile Vortex.

Another study found NiTi had superior fatigue life for ProTaper Gold (Dentsply Tulsa Dental) and ProTaper Universal (Dentsply Tulsa Dental) run in a water bath at room temperature.[82] However, recently Vasconcelos and colleagues[83] used a water bath to maintain temperature at 20°C and 37°C to test the fatigue life of rotary instruments at body temperature. They found that at 20°C, Hyflex CM showed the highest resistance to fracture, whereas ProTaper Universal showed the lowest resistance to fracture. At 37°C, resistance to fatigue fracture was significantly reduced, up to 85%, for all tested instruments: HyFlex CM, Vortex Blue, TRUShape, and, to a lesser extent, ProTaper Universal.

Autoclave cycle effects on flexural fatigue have also been studied,[87–89] with varying results. One study found that autoclave sterilization resulted in an increase of 39% in the remaining number of cycles to failure,[87] whereas other investigators found a significant increase only for K3XF files.[89] This finding varies from data that showed a reduction of mean cycles to failure for 25/.06 TF after repeated autoclaving, whereas 25/.04 TF and both GT Series X files tested were not significantly affected.[88]

## Corrosion

NiTi alloys exhibit a high intrinsic corrosion resistance because of the thermodynamic stability of Ni and the low degree of disorder in a thin protective Ti-dioxide layer. Although there is no specific concern about corrosion during single-patient use, reprocessing may be associated with material deterioration by electrochemical processes.[90–95]

A study[96] evaluated the pitting corrosion resistance of NiTi rotary instruments with different surface treatments in ethylenediaminetetraacetic acid (EDTA) and sodium chloride solutions. NiTi files with physical vapor deposition coating and electropolishing surface treatments showed an increased corrosion resistance.

Fayyad and Mahran[95] compared the effect of 5.25% sodium hypochlorite (NaOCl) or 17% EDTA on the surface topography and roughness of GTX, TF, RaCe, and Hero Shaper (MicroMega) instruments using atomic force microscopy. They found that 5.25% NaOCl increased the surface roughness of TF and Hero Shaper significantly compared with RaCe and GTX instruments.

The effect of irrigation solutions and other environments on heat-treated instruments with an oxide coating is currently unknown. As this has potential implications on wear resistance and cutting ability, more research is needed in this regard to guide decision-making; it should be mentioned that some of the recently introduced instruments are specifically marketed as single-patient-use devices.

## CLINICAL USE AND OUTCOMES

Another major innovation introduced in the last years is reciprocation action, rather than continuous rotation.[6] This innovation has resulted in specifically designed instruments (WaveOne, WaveOne Gold, Dentsply Maillefer; Reciproc, Reciproc Blue, VDW, Munich, Germany). The reported shaping ability, based on micro-CT studies, similar to other NiTi instruments that are used in continuous rotation. Special electric motors are needed for reciprocation action, with defined presets for angles, speed, and torque. One motor system is promoted as adaptive, changing from continuous rotation to reciprocation motion when a certain torque threshold is reached.

A common thread for all relevant innovation described earlier is that actual clinical outcome data are sparse, which is also true for NiTi rotary root canal preparation in general. Only Cheung and Chiu[2] retrospectively compared root canal treatment with stainless steel files and NiTi rotaries, which significantly better periapical outcomes for the latter. Pain as a patient-reported outcome was considered in the context of rotary instrumentation.[97] In that prospective study patients seen by a single clinician experienced more pain, both in numbers of incidences and in intensity, when hand instrumentation only was performed compared by those that had canals shaped with a rotary system. For recently introduced rotary instruments, one report described the immediate postoperative course for patients after root canal treatment with or without the use of a mechanical glide path file. In another prospective study on the effect of mechanized glide path preparation reported pain, and the use of analgesics, higher when K-files were used compared with NiTi path files.[98]

In summary, current innovation exists with changes in instrument design, some of them substantial, whereas others are rather discrete. A more relevant change is occurring in manufacturing processes, with various proprietary heat treatments generating rotaries with completely different properties. In vitro testing is ongoing and, because of the lack of consistent methodology gives only some guidelines for clinical use. Lastly, clinical data are lacking for many current instruments; therefore, it is not clear if improvements in flexibility and resistance to fatigue will translate to better outcomes. Current and future developments of instruments and strategies should aim at providing antibiofilm effects less radicular structure to preserve structural strength with the intention to serve the ultimate goal, long-term retention of the natural dentition.

## REFERENCES

1. Peters OA, Barbakow F, Peters CI. An analysis of endodontic treatment with three nickel-titanium rotary root canal preparation techniques. Int Endod J 2004;37(12): 849–59.

2. Cheung GS, Liu CS. A retrospective study of endodontic treatment outcome between nickel-titanium rotary and stainless steel hand filing techniques. J Endod 2009;35(7):938–43.

3. Shen Y, Zhou HM, Zheng YF, et al. Current challenges and concepts of the thermomechanical treatment of nickel-titanium instruments. J Endod 2013;39(2): 163–72.

4. Plotino G, Ahmed HM, Grande NM, et al. Current assessment of reciprocation in endodontic preparation: a comprehensive review–part II: properties and effectiveness. J Endod 2015;41(12):1939–50.

5. Hülsmann M, Peters OA, Dummer PMH. Mechanical preparation of root canals: shaping goals, techniques and means. Endod Top 2005;10:30–76.

6. Yared G. Canal preparation using only one Ni-Ti rotary instrument: preliminary observations. Int Endod J 2008;41(4):339–44.

7. Perez-Higueras JJ, Arias A, de la Macorra JC. Cyclic fatigue resistance of K3, K3XF, and twisted file nickel-titanium files under continuous rotation or reciprocating motion. J Endod 2013;39(12):1585–8.

8. Koch J, Borg J, Mattson A, et al. An in vitro comparative study of intracanal fluid motion and wall shear stress induced by ultrasonic and polymer rotary finishing files in a simulated root canal model. ISRN Dent 2012;2012:764041.

9. Peters OA, Schönenberger K, Laib A. Effects of four Ni-Ti preparation techniques on root canal geometry assessed by micro computed tomography. Int Endod J 2001;34(3):221–30.

10. Metzger Z, Teperovich E, Zary R, et al. The self-adjusting file (SAF). Part 1: respecting the root canal anatomy–a new concept of endodontic files and its implementation. J Endod 2010;36(4):679–90.

11. Ng YL, Mann V, Gulabivala K. A prospective study of the factors affecting outcomes of nonsurgical root canal treatment: part 1: periapical health. Int Endod J 2011;44(7):583–609.

12. Ng YL, Mann V, Gulabivala K. A prospective study of the factors affecting outcomes of non-surgical root canal treatment: part 2: tooth survival. Int Endod J 2011;44(7):610–25.

13. Reeh ES, Messer HH, Douglas WH. Reduction in tooth stiffness as a result of endodontic and restorative procedures. J Endod 1989;15(11):512–6.

14. Krishan R, Paqué F, Ossareh A, et al. Impacts of conservative endodontic cavity on root canal instrumentation efficacy and resistance to fracture assessed in incisors, premolars, and molars. J Endod 2014;40(8):1160–6.

15. Lang H, Korkmaz Y, Schneider K, et al. Impact of endodontic treatments on the rigidity of the root. J Dent Res 2006;85(4):364–8.

16. Zelic K, Vukicevic A, Jovicic G, et al. Mechanical weakening of devitalized teeth: three dimensional finite element analysis and prediction of tooth fracture. Int Endod J 2015;48(9):850–63.
17. Gluskin AH, Peters CI, Peters OA. Minimally invasive endodontics: challenging prevailing paradigms. Br Dent J 2014;216(6):347–53.
18. Rzhanov EA, Belyeva TS. Design features of rotary root canal instruments. ENDO (Lond) 2012;6(1):29–39.
19. Sanghvi Z, Mistry K. Design features of rotary instruments in endodontics. J Ahmedabad Dent Coll 2011;2(1):6–11.
20. Grande NM, Plotino G, Butti A, et al. Modern endodontic NiTi systems: morphological and technical characteristics. Part I: "new generation" Ni-Ti systems. Endod Ther 2005;5(1):11–6.
21. Mize SB, Clement DJ, Pruett JP, et al. Effect of sterilization on cyclic fatigue of rotary nickel-titanium endodontic instruments. J Endod 1998;24(12):843–7.
22. Mizutani T, Ohno N, Nakamura H. Anatomical study of the root apex in the maxillary anterior teeth. J Endod 1992;18(7):344–7.
23. Roane JB. Principles of preparation using the balanced force technique. In: Hardin J, editor. Clark's clinical dentistry, vol. 4. Philadelphia: JB Lippincott Co; 1991. p. 1–39.
24. Diemer F, Michetti J, Mallet J, et al. Effect of asymmetry on the behavior of prototype rotary triple helix root canal instruments. J Endod 2013;39(6):829–32.
25. Peters OA, Arias A, Paqué F. A micro–computed tomographic assessment of root canal preparation with a novel instrument, TRUShape, in mesial roots of mandibular molars. J Endod 2015;41(9):1445–50.
26. Peters OA, Boessler C, Paqué F. Root canal preparation with a novel nickel-titanium instrument evaluated with micro-computed tomography: canal surface preparation over time. J Endod 2010;36(6):1068–72.
27. Otsuka K, Wayman C. Mechanism of shape memory effect and superelasticity. In: Press CU, editor. Shape memory alloys. 1st edition. Cambridge (United Kingdom): 1998. p. 27–48.
28. Thompson SA. An overview of nickel-titanium alloys used in dentistry. Int Endod J 2000;33(4):297–310.
29. Otsuka K, Ren X. Physical metallurgy of Ti-Ni-based shape memory alloys. Prog Mater Sci 2005;50:511–678.
30. Saburi T. Shape memory alloys. In: Press CU, editor. Shape memory alloys. 1st edition. Cambridge (United Kingdom): 1998. p. 49–96.
31. Miyazaki S, Ohmi Y, Otsuka K, et al. Characteristics of deformation and transformation pseudoelasticity in Ti-Ni alloys. J Phys 1982;43(4):255–60.
32. Tang W. Thermodynamic study of the low-temperature phase B19' and the martensitic transformation in near-equiatomic Ti-Ni shape memory alloys. Metall Mater Trans 1997;28A:537–44.
33. Kuhn G, Jordan L. Fatigue and mechanical properties of nickel-titanium endodontic instruments. J Endod 2002;28(10):716–20.
34. Hayashi Y, Yoneyama T, Yahata Y, et al. Phase transformation behaviour and bending properties of hybrid nickel-titanium rotary endodontic instruments. Int Endod J 2007;40(4):247–53.
35. Yahata Y, Yoneyama T, Hayashi Y, et al. Effect of heat treatment on transformation temperatures and bending properties of nickel-titanium endodontic instruments. Int Endod J 2009;42(7):621–6.

36. Alapati S, Brantley W, Lijima M, et al. Micro-XRD and temperature modulated DSC investigation of nickel-titanium rotary endodontic instruments. Dent Mater 2009;25(10):1221–9.

37. Braga L, Buono V, Bahia M. Impact of heat treatments on the fatigue resistance of different rotary nickel-titanium instruments. J Endod 2014;40(9):1494–7.

38. Peixoto I, Pereira E, Silva J, et al. Flexural fatigue and torsional resistance of ProFile GT and ProFile GT series X instruments. J Endod 2010;36(4):741–4.

39. Shen Y, Zhou H, Zheng Y, et al. Metallurgical characterization of controlled memory wire nickel-titanium rotary instruments. J Endod 2011;37(11):1566–71.

40. Braga L, Magalhães R, Nakagawa R, et al. Physical and mechanical properties of twisted or ground nickel-titanium instruments. Int Endod J 2013;46(5):458–65.

41. Pereira E, Peixoto I, Viana A, et al. Physical and mechanical properties of a thermomechanically treated NiTi wire used in the manufacture of rotary endodontic instruments. Int Endod J 2012;45(5):469–74.

42. Ye J, Gao Y. Metallurgical characterization of M-wire nickel-titanium shape memory alloy used for endodontic rotary instruments during low-cycle fatigue. J Endod 2012;38(7):105–7.

43. Pruett J, Clement D, Carnes D. Cyclic fatigue testing of titanium endodontic instruments. J Endod 1997;23(2):77–85.

44. Pereira E, Gomes R, Leroy A, et al. Mechanical behavior of M-Wire and conventional NiTi wire used to manufacture rotary endodontic instruments. Dent Mater 2013;29(12):e318–24.

45. Berendt C, Yang J. Endodontic instruments with improved fatigue resistance. International Conference on Shape Memory and Superelastic Technologies. Pacific Grove (CA), May 7, 2006.

46. Johnson E, Lloyd A, Kuttler S, et al. Comparison between a novel nickel-titanium alloy and 508 nitinol on the cyclic fatigue life of ProFile 25/.04 rotary instruments. J Endod 2008;34(11):1406–9.

47. Berendt C. Method of preparing nitinol for use in manufacturing instruments with improved fatigue resistance. Inventor; Sportswire, L.L.C., assignee; 2007.

48. Miyazaki S, Otsuka K. Deformation and transition behaviour associated with the R-phase in Ti-Ni alloys. Metall Trans A 1986;17A:54–63.

49. Larsen C, Watanabe I, Glickman G, et al. Cyclic fatigue analysis of a new generation of nickel-titanium rotary instruments. J Endod 2009;35(3):401–3.

50. Al-Hadlaq S, Aljarbou F, AlThumairy R. Evaluation of cyclic flexural fatigue of M-wire nickel-titanium rotary instruments. J Endod 2010;36(2):305–7.

51. Gao Y, Shotton V, Wilkinson K, et al. Effects of raw material and rotational speed on the cyclic fatigue of ProFile Vortex rotary instruments. J Endod 2010;36(7):1205–9.

52. Miyai K, Ebihara A, Hayashi Y, et al. Influence of phase transformation on the torsional and bending properties of nickel-titanium rotary endodontic instruments. Int Endod J 2006;39(2):119–26.

53. Ebihara A, Yahata Y, Miyara K, et al. Heat treatment of nickel-titanium rotary endodontic instruments: effects on bending properties and shaping abilities. Int Endod J 2011;44(9):843–9.

54. Kell T, Azarpazhooh A, Peters O, et al. Torsional profiles of new and used 20/.06 GT series X and GT rotary endodontic instruments. J Endod 2009;35(9):1278–81.

55. Rodrigues R, Lopes H, Elias C, et al. Influence of different manufacturing methods on the cyclic fatigue of rotary nickel-titanium endodontic instruments. Int Endod J 2011;37(11):1553–7.

56. Shen Y, Riyahi A, Campbell L, et al. Effect of a combination of torsional and cyclic fatigue preloading on the fracture behavior of K3 and K3XF instruments. J Endod 2015;41(4):526–30.

57. Kim H, Yum J, Hur B, et al. Cyclic fatigue and fracture characteristics of ground and twisted nickel-titanium rotary files. J Endod 2010;36(1):147–52.

58. Gambarini G, Gerosa R, De Luca M, et al. Mechanical properties of a new and improved nickel-titanium alloy for endodontic use: an evaluation of the flexibility. Oral Surg Oral Med Oral Pathol Oral Radiol Endod 2008;105(6):798–800.

59. Pirani C, Iacono F, Generali L, et al. HyFlex EDM: superficial features, metallurgical analysis and fatigue resistance of innovative electro discharge machined NiTi rotary instruments. Int Endod J 2016;49(5):483–93.

60. Gutmann J, Gao Y. Alteration in the inherent metallic and surface properties of nickel-titanium root canal instruments to enhance performance, durability and safety: a focused review. Int Endod J 2012;45(2):113–28.

61. Santos L, Bahia M, Las Casas E, et al. Comparison of the mechanical behavior between controlled memory and superelastic nickel-titanium files via finite element analysis. J Endod 2013;39(11):1444–7.

62. Pereira E, Viana A, Buono V, et al. Behavior of nickel-titanium instruments manufactured with different thermal treatments. J Endod 2015;41(11):67–71.

63. Hornbogen H. Fatigue of copper-based shape memory alloys. In: Butterworth H, editor. Engineering aspects of shape memory alloys. London: 1990. p. 267-82.

64. Peters O, Gluskin A, Weiss R, et al. An in vitro assessment of the physical properties of novel Hyflex nickel-titanium rotary instruments. Int Endod J 2012;45(11):1027–34.

65. Shen Y, Qian W, Abtin H, et al. Effect of environment on fatigue failure of controlled memory wire nickel-titanium rotary instruments. J Endod 2012;38(3):376–80.

66. Shen Y, Oian W, Abtin H, et al. Fatigue testing of controlled memory wire nickel-titanium rotary instruments. J Endod 2011;37(7):997–1001.

67. Campbell L, Shen Y, Zhou H, et al. Effect of fatigue on torsional failure of nickel-titanium controlled memory instruments. J Endod 2014;40(4):562–5.

68. Wycoff R, Berzins D. An in vitro comparison of torsional stress properties of three different rotary nickel-titanium files with a similar cross-sectional design. J Endod 2012;38(8):1118–20.

69. Zhu QG, Fang M, Shen GQ, et al. Effects of manipulation on mechanical properties of cervical and degree of fatigue in patients with cervical spondylosis. Zhongguo Gu Shang 2012;25(1):18–21 [in Chinese].

70. Yum J, Cheung G, Park J, et al. Torsional strength and toughness of nickel-titanium rotary files. J Endod 2008;37(3):382–6.

71. Ninan E, Berzins D. Torsional and bending properties of shape memory and superelastic nickel-titanium rotary instruments. J Endod 2013;39(1):101–4.

72. Sattapan B, Nervo G, Palamara J, et al. Defects in rotary nickel-titanium files after clinical use. J Endod 2000;26(3):161–5.

73. Haikel Y, Serfaty R, Bateman G, et al. Dynamic and cyclic fatigue of engine-driven rotary nickel-titanium endodontic instruments. J Endod 1999;25(6):434–40.

74. Bahia M, Buono V. Decrease in fatigue resistance of nickel-titanium rotary instruments after clinical use in curved root canals. Oral Surg Oral Med Oral Pathol Oral Radiol Endod 2005;100(2):249–55.

75. Câmara A, Aguiar C, De Figueiredo J. Evaluation of the root dentine cutting effectiveness of the HERO 642, HERO Apical, and HERO Shaper rotary systems. Aust Endod J 2008;34(3):94–100.

76. Schäfer E, Oitzinger M. Cutting efficiency of five different types of rotary nickel-titanium instruments. J Endod 2008;34(2):198–200.

77. Boessler C, Paqué F, Peters O. The effect of electropolishing on torque and force during simulated root canal preparation with ProTaper shaping files. J Endod 2009;35(1):102–6.

78. Morgental R, Vier-Pelisser F, Kopper P, et al. Cutting efficiency of conventional and martensitic nickel-titanium instruments for coronal flaring. J Endod 2013; 39(12):1634–8.

79. Peixoto I, Pereira E, Aun D, et al. Constant insertion rate methodology of measuring torque and apical force in 3 nickel-titanium instruments with different cross-sectional designs. J Endod 2015;41(9):1540–4.

80. Seago S, Bergeron B, Kirkpatrick T, et al. Effect of repeated simulated clinical use and sterilization on the cutting efficiency and flexibility of Hyflex CM nickel-titanium rotary files. J Endod 2015;41(5):725–8.

81. Plotino G, Grande N, Cotti E, et al. Blue treatment enhances cyclic fatigue resistance of Vortex nickel-titanium rotary files. J Endod 2014;40(9):1451–3.

82. Hieawy A, Haapasalo M, Zhou H, et al. Phase transformation behavior and resistance to bending and cyclic fatigue of ProTaper Gold and ProTaper Universal instruments. J Endod 2015;41(7):1134–8.

83. Vasconcelos R, Murphy S, Carvalho C, et al. Evidence for reduced fatigue resistance of contemporary rotary instruments exposed to body temperature. J Endod 2016;42(5):82–7.

84. Melo M, Bahia M, Buono V. Fatigue resistance of engine-driven rotary nickel-titanium endodontic instruments. J Endod 2002;28(11):765–9.

85. Capar I, Kaval M, Ertas H, et al. Comparison of the cyclic fatigue resistance of 5 different rotary pathfinding instruments made of nickel-titanium wire, M-Wire, and controlled memory wire. J Endod 2015;41(4):535–8.

86. Gao Y, Gutmann JL, Wilkinson K, et al. Evaluation of the impact of raw materials on the fatigue and mechanical properties of ProFile Vortex rotary instruments. J Endod 2012;38(3):398–401.

87. Viana A, Gonzalez B, Buono V, et al. Influence of sterilization on mechanical properties and fatigue resistance of nickel-titanium rotary endodontic instruments. Int Endod J 2006;39(9):709–15.

88. Hilfer P, Bergeron B, Mayerchak M, et al. Multiple autoclave cycle effects on cyclic fatigue of nickel-titanium rotary files produced by new manufacturing methods. J Endod 2011;37(1):72–4.

89. Plotino G, Constanzo A, Grande N, et al. Experimental evaluation on the influence of autoclave sterilization on the cyclic fatigue of new nickel-titanium rotary instruments. J Endod 2012;38(2):222–5.

90. Kassab E, Neelakantan L, Frotscher M, et al. Effect of ternary element addition on the corrosion behaviour of NiTi shape memory alloys. Mater Corrosion 2014; 65(1):18–22.

91. Sonntag D, Peters O. Effect of prion decontamination protocols on nickel-titanium rotary surfaces. J Endod 2007;33(4):442–6.

92. Bonaccorso A, Schäffer E, Condorelli G, et al. Chemical analysis of nickel-titanium rotary instruments with and without electropolishing after cleaning procedures with sodium hypochlorite. J Endod 2008;34(11):1391–5.

93. Pedullà E, Franciosi G, Ounsi H, et al. Cyclic fatigue resistance of nickel-titanium instruments after immersion in irrigant solutions with or without surfactants. J Endod 2014;40(8):1245–9.

94. Pedullà E, Grande N, Plotino G, et al. Cyclic fatigue resistance of two reciprocating nickel-titanium instruments after immersion in sodium hypochlorite. Int Endod J 2013;46(2):155–9.

95. Fayyard D, Mahran A. Atomic force microscopic evaluation of nanostructure alterations of rotary NiTi instruments after immersion in irrigating solutions. Int Endod J 2014;47(6):567–73.

96. Bonaccorso A, Cantatore G, Condorelli G, et al. Shaping ability of four nickel-titanium rotary instruments in simulated S-shaped canals. Int Endod J 2009;35: 883–6.

97. Arias A, Macorra JC, Azabal M, et al. Prospective case controlled clinical study of post-endodontic pain after rotary root canal preparation performed by a single operator. J Dent 2015;43(3):389–95.

98. Pasqualini D, Mollo L, Scotti N, et al. Postoperative pain after manual and mechanical glide path: a randomized clinical trial. J Endod 2012;38(1):32–6.

# Endodontic Treatment Outcomes

Nadia Chugal, DDS, MS, MPH[a],*, Sanjay M. Mallya, MDS, PhD[b], Bill Kahler, DClinDent, PhD[c],
Louis M. Lin, BDS, DMD, PhD[d]

## KEYWORDS

- Root canal treatment • Success and failure • Endodontics • Treatment outcome
- Endodontic prognosis • Healing • Mature teeth • Immature teeth

## KEY POINTS

- Primary goals of endodontic treatment of mature and immature permanent teeth are prevention and/or elimination of apical periodontitis and resolution of patient symptoms.
- Additional treatment specific goals are described for treatment of immature teeth with vital and/or necrotic pulps.
- Robust criteria for outcome assessment are an essential determinant for any measure of treatment success for both mature and immature teeth.
- Assessment of endodontic treatment outcomes has evolved from disease-based criteria to patient-centered values emphasizing survival and function even in the presence of inflammatory periapical disease.
- Disease-free treatment outcome should always be the goal of all endodontic treatments.

## INTRODUCTION

Outcome assessment of endodontically treated teeth has been extensively studied. The terminology used to assess outcomes is varied and may be confusing to practicing dentists. The knowledge gained from the outcome studies should be applied to the case assessment before the commencement of endodontic treatment. This information must be part of preoperative discussion, treatment planning, and informed consent.

Disclosure: Authors disclose no conflict of interest.
Portions of this text are from: Chugal N, Mallya SM, Kahler B. Criteria for outcome assessment of non-surgical endodontic treatment. In: Chugal N, Lin LM, editors. Endodontic prognosis: clinical guide for optimal treatment outcome. 1st edition. Springer International Publishing Switzerland, 2017. With permission of Springer.
[a] Section of Endodontics, UCLA School of Dentistry, CHS A3-075, 10833 Le Conte Avenue, Los Angeles, CA 90095-1668, USA; [b] Section of Oral and Maxillofacial Radiology, UCLA School of Dentistry, CHS 53-068B, Los Angeles, CA 90095-1668, USA; [c] School of Dentistry, The University of Queensland Oral Health Centre, 288 Herston Road, Corner Bramston Terrace & Herston Road, Herston, Queensland 4006, Australia; [d] Department of Endodontics, New York University College of Dentistry, 345 East 24th Street, New York, NY 10010, USA
* Corresponding author.
*E-mail address:* nchugal@dentistry.ucla.edu

Methods used to evaluate the outcome of endodontic therapy include clinical examination for resolution of clinical symptoms and signs, radiographic evaluation of periapical osseous status, and histopathologic findings of biopsy specimens. Symptoms include spontaneous pain and/or pain to percussion, palpation, and biting after endodontic treatment and decrease to minimal levels by 7 days after root canal treatment.[1] Persistent pain may be from nonodontogenic causes[2] or persistent infection.[3] The signs include swelling or draining sinus tract after endodontic treatment.[3–5]

A landmark study on endodontic outcome assessment by Strindberg laid the foundation for conduct of future endodontic outcome studies.[6] The highlights of this study are that it

1. Established criteria for evaluation of endodontic outcome, commonly referred to as Strindberg criteria
2. Arrived at outcome rates for orthograde (conventional) endodontic treatment
3. Related the outcome of endodontic treatment to the preoperative periapical diagnosis
4. Defined the duration and frequency of follow-up: every 6 months for the first 2 years and yearly thereafter up to a minimum of 4 years postoperatively

The evaluation of the result of therapy was based on comparative analysis of clinical presentation and radiographic evaluation of the treated tooth at the time of treatment and follow-up examination. Determination of endodontic outcome was expressed as "success," "failure," or "uncertain" and became known as Strindberg criteria.

## STRINDBERG CRITERIA
### Success

Clinical
- No symptoms

Radiographic
- Contours and width of periodontal ligament are normal (**Fig. 1**).

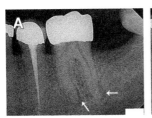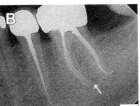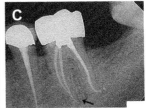

**Fig. 1.** Strindberg criteria for success: re-establishment of the normal apical periodontal structures. (*A*) Pretreatment periapical radiograph demonstrating widening of the periodontal ligament space and loss of the adjacent lamina dura around the mesial and distal roots of the mandibular first molar (*white arrows*). (*B*) Periapical radiographs made after the completion of endodontic treatment. Trabecular bone around the mesial root apex is slightly radiolucent (*white arrow*), and the bony contours of the lamina dura are not established around the root apex. Note reduction of radiolucency around the distal root apex. (*C*) Follow-up periapical radiograph taken at the 1-year recall visit. Trabecular bone around both roots is of normal density. The lamina dura around both root apices is also formed (*black arrow*). (*Courtesy of* Dr Charles Maupin. *From* Chugal N, Mallya SM, Kahler B. Criteria for outcome assessment of non-surgical endodontic treatment. In: Chugal N, Lin LM, editors. Endodontic prognosis: clinical guide for optimal treatment outcome. 1st edition. Springer International Publishing Switzerland, 2017. With permission of Springer.)

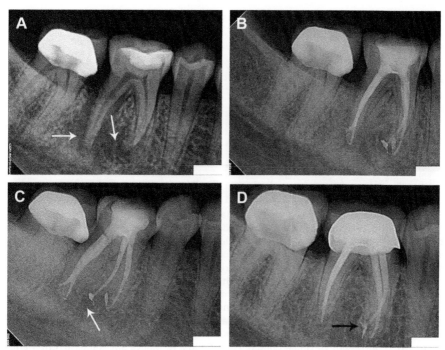

**Fig. 2.** Strindberg criteria for success: altered periodontal ligament space contours around excess endodontic material/root filling. (*A*) Pretreatment periapical radiograph demonstrating an irregular radiolucency that encompasses almost the entire length of the distal root and the apex of the mesial root (*white arrows*). Note multiple mesial roots and pulp canals. (*B, C*) Periapical radiographs made at the completion of endodontic obturation after 4 months of dressing with calcium hydroxide. The radiographs were taken with different horizontal angulation to separate the buccal and lingual pulp canals in the 2 roots. Note persistence of the radiolucency around the mesial root apex (*white arrow*) but considerable resolution with partial osseous healing around the distal root. (*D*) Follow-up periapical radiograph made at a recall visit 3.5 years after completion of endodontic therapy. Trabecular bone around both roots is of normal density. The lamina dura around both root apices is also formed. Minimal widening of the periodontal ligament space is seen adjacent to the excess endodontic filling material (*black arrow*). (*Courtesy of* Dr Charles Maupin. *From* Chugal N, Mallya SM, Kahler B. Criteria for outcome assessment of non-surgical endodontic treatment. In: Chugal N, Lin LM, editors. Endodontic prognosis: clinical guide for optimal treatment outcome. 1st edition. Springer International Publishing Switzerland, 2017. With permission of Springer.)

- Periodontal ligament contours are widened mainly around excess root filling (**Fig. 2**).
- Lamina dura is intact (**Figs. 3** and **4**).

### Failure

Clinical
- Symptoms present

Radiographic
- Unchanged periradicular rarefaction (**Fig. 5**)
- Decrease in periradicular rarefaction but no resolution (**Fig. 6**)
- Appearance of new rarefaction or an increase in the size of initial rarefaction (**Fig. 7**)
- Discontinuous or poorly defined lamina dura

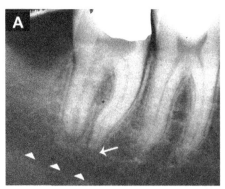
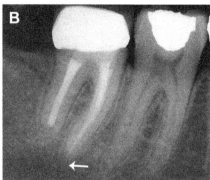

**Fig. 3.** Strindberg criteria for success: normal lamina dura. (*A*) Pretreatment periapical radiograph showing disruption of lamina dura and widening of the periodontal ligament space around the mesial root apex of the mandibular second molar (*white arrow*) and resorption in the distal root canal. An incidental finding is the proximity of the root apices to the mandibular canal lumen (*arrowheads*). (*B*) Periapical radiographs made 1 year after completion of endodontic treatment, after 15 months and 2 exchanges of calcium hydroxide dressing. Note normal trabecular architecture around mesial root apex with an intact lamina dura (*white arrow*). The distal root is shortened but with normal architecture of the adjacent trabecular bone, suggestive of arrested resorption. As described in Strindberg's original article, teeth with root resorption but no periradicular pathologic changes are categorized as success. (*Courtesy of* Dr Nadia Chugal. *From* Chugal N, Mallya SM, Kahler B. Criteria for outcome assessment of non-surgical endodontic treatment. In: Chugal N, Lin LM, editors. Endodontic prognosis: clinical guide for optimal treatment outcome. 1st edition. Springer International Publishing Switzerland, 2017. With permission of Springer.)

### Uncertain

Radiographic
- Ambiguous or technically unsatisfactory radiograph that could not be interpreted with certainty (**Fig. 8**)
- Periradicular rarefaction less than 1 mm and disrupted lamina dura
- Tooth extracted prior to recall due to reasons not related to endodontic outcome

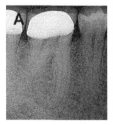
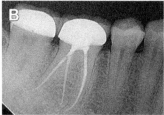
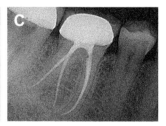

**Fig. 4.** Strindberg criteria for success: normal lamina dura. (*A*) Pretreatment periapical radiograph showing a mandibular molar with 3 roots. The periodontal ligament space around all roots is discernible. (*B, C*) Periapical radiographs made immediately after obturation and 1 year after completion of endodontic treatment. Note that there are no interval changes in the periodontal structures. (*Courtesy of* Dr Charles Maupin. *From* Chugal N, Mallya SM, Kahler B. Criteria for outcome assessment of non-surgical endodontic treatment. In: Chugal N, Lin LM, editors. Endodontic prognosis: clinical guide for optimal treatment outcome. 1st edition. Springer International Publishing Switzerland, 2017. With permission of Springer.)

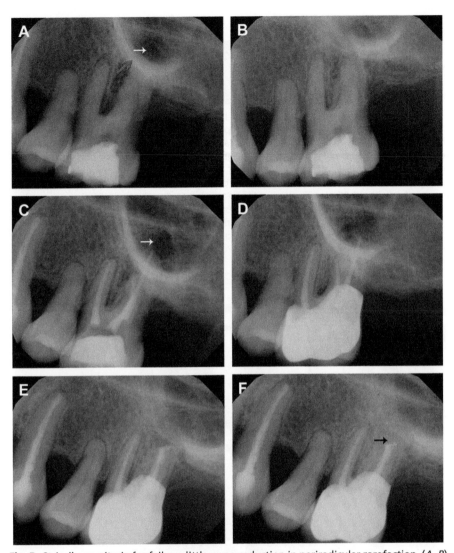

**Fig. 5.** Strindberg criteria for failure: little or no reduction in periradicular rarefaction. (*A, B*) Pretreatment periapical radiograph showing a periapical radiolucency around the palatal root of the maxillary first molar (*white arrow*). Note the superimposition of the zygomatic process of the maxilla (*red arrow*) that can be avoided by changing the vertical angulation as in panel b. (*C, D*) Follow-up periapical radiographs after completion of endodontic treatment show persistence of the periapical radiolucency (*white arrow*). Nine months after completion of endodontic treatment, the tooth became symptomatic again. The AAE classification categorizes this radiographic appearance as "nonhealed" (symptomatic). (*E, F*) Periapical radiographs made 1 year after surgical management of the palatal root of the maxillary first molar. Note complete resolution and osseous healing around the palatal root (*black arrow*). (*Courtesy of* Dr Alexis Moore and Dr David Han. *From* Chugal N, Mallya SM, Kahler B. Criteria for outcome assessment of non-surgical endodontic treatment. In: Chugal N, Lin LM, editors. Endodontic prognosis: clinical guide for optimal treatment outcome. 1st edition. Springer International Publishing Switzerland, 2017. With permission of Springer.)

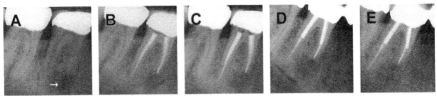

**Fig. 6.** Strindberg criteria for failure: decrease in size but no resolution of periradicular rarefaction. (*A*) Pretreatment periapical radiograph showing a periapical radiolucency around the mesial root of the mandibular first molar (*arrow*). Note external resorption of the mesial root apex. (*B–E*) Sequential periapical radiographs after completion of endodontic treatment show an increase in the radiodensity of the periapical bone. The area of rarefaction is persistent, however, and in the appropriate clinical context may be categorized as a treatment failure. The AAE classification categorizes this as "nonhealed" (if symptomatic) or "healing" (if clinically asymptomatic). (*Courtesy of* Dr Nadia Chugal. *From* Chugal N, Mallya SM, Kahler B. Criteria for outcome assessment of non-surgical endodontic treatment. In: Chugal N, Lin LM, editors. Endodontic prognosis: clinical guide for optimal treatment outcome. 1st edition. Springer International Publishing Switzerland, 2017. With permission of Springer.)

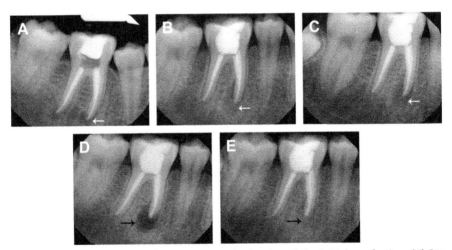

**Fig. 7.** Strindberg criteria for failure: Increase in the size of the initial rarefaction. (*A*) Pretreatment periapical radiograph showing disruption of lamina dura and widening of the periodontal ligament space around the root apices of the mandibular first molar, particularly evident around the mesial root (*white arrow*). The surrounding trabecular bone is sclerotic, suggestive of a chronic inflammatory process. (*B, C*) Follow-up periapical radiographs 3.5 years after completion of endodontic treatment show persistence and an increase in the size of the periapical radiolucency (*white arrow*) and in the appropriate clinical context (accompanied with increasing clinical symptoms of pain) is categorized as a treatment failure. (*D*) Periapical radiograph made after completion of endodontic surgery. Note radiolucent bony defect around the mesial root apex (*black arrow*). (*E*) Osseous healing and resolution of the periapical radiolucency (*black arrow*). (*Courtesy of* Dr David Han. *From* Chugal N, Mallya SM, Kahler B. Criteria for outcome assessment of non-surgical endodontic treatment. In: Chugal N, Lin LM, editors. Endodontic prognosis: clinical guide for optimal treatment outcome. 1st edition. Springer International Publishing Switzerland, 2017. With permission of Springer.)

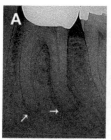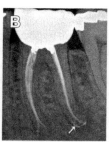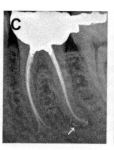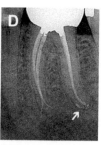

**Fig. 8.** Strindberg criteria, uncertain outcome: periapical rarefaction less than 1 mm and with broken lamina dura. (*A*) Pretreatment periapical radiograph showing periradicular rarefaction around the mesial and distal roots of the mandibular first molar (*white arrows*). (*B*) Periapical radiograph made immediately after obturation, after 4 months in calcium hydroxide intracanal dressing. Note reduction in periapical radiolucency during this 4-month period. Slight excess of endodontic filling material is noted at the distal root apex (*white arrow*). (*C*) Periapical radiograph made at 6 months postobturation. The periodontal ligament space at the distal root apex is wide (*white arrow*), with absence of the lamina dura. As an asymptomatic tooth, this radiographic appearance is categorized as an uncertain endodontic outcome. In contrast, the AAE classification categorizes this as "healing" (clinically asymptomatic). (*D*) Periapical radiograph made 18 months post-treatment. The periodontal ligament space at the distal root apex is minimally wide. Note presence of an intact lamina dura around the root (*white arrow*) signifying resolved periapical radiolucency and a successful radiographic outcome. The AAE classification categorizes this as "healed" and "functional" (clinically asymptomatic). (*Courtesy of* Dr Charles Maupin. *From* Chugal N, Mallya SM, Kahler B. Criteria for outcome assessment of non-surgical endodontic treatment. In: Chugal N, Lin LM, editors. Endodontic prognosis: clinical guide for optimal treatment outcome. 1st edition. Springer International Publishing Switzerland, 2017. With permission of Springer.)

These criteria were accepted as a standard by which the outcome of endodontically treated teeth are evaluated and continue to be widely used. It became evident that Strindberg criteria were rigid. For example, only teeth with complete absence of clinical signs and symptoms and normal radiographic presentation are classified as "success" (see **Figs. 1–3**). In contrast, an asymptomatic tooth with the appearance of broken or poorly defined lamina dura is classified as uncertain (see **Fig. 8**), and clinical judgment is required for its subsequent management.

## VARIABILITY OF RADIOGRAPHIC INTERPRETATION

Absence of clinical symptoms and periapical radiolucency are currently the principal outcome measures that denote successful endodontic treatment. Radiographic examination, however, has its limitations. Radiographs provide a static image of the degree of mineralization in the tooth and its surrounding periodontal structures. For changes in bone to be radiographically apparent, there must be sufficient demineralization (or remineralization) within the lesion. A classic study examined the sensitivity of conventional radiography to detect experimental lesions in bone and showed that periapical lesions confined to the cancellous bone are not predictably detected.[7] Furthermore, radiographic evaluations tend to be subjective and influenced by observer bias.[4,8,9] These data underscore the need to calibrate evaluators and minimize inconsistencies in radiographic evaluation when designing studies evaluating endodontic treatment outcomes. Importantly, the inherent observer variability in radiographic analyses emphasizes the need to select those radiographic outcome measures that are robust to be used in clinical practice.

## THE PERIAPICAL INDEX SCORING SYSTEM

In clinical practice, the principal endpoints to assess endodontic treatment outcomes are clinical findings and the status of apical periodontal bone as assessed by periapical radiography. These radiographic assessments are based on subjective evaluation of changes in radiodensity of the periapical lesion with osseous healing and with the reestablishment of the apical periodontal structures. Currently used criteria for endodontic outcomes assessment are Strindberg criteria and the American Association of Endodontics (AAE) classification, and both of these require radiographic assessment as one of the key endpoints analyzed.

For widespread application of such criteria, clinicians should be trained to reproducibly identify radiographic features of apical periodontitis. Equally important, research studies that examine endodontic treatment outcomes should use reliable and reproducible criteria to define success and failure. To address this issue, a scoring system for apical periodontitis, as depicted on conventional 2-D periapical radiographs, was developed.[10] This scale provides clinicians and researchers with a reliable and reproducible tool to assess endodontic outcomes and to reasonably discriminate between subpoulations of success and failure.

The periapical index (PAI) is a structured scoring system for categorization of radiographic features of apical periodontitis. It is based on a visual scale of periapical periodontitis severity and was built on a classic study of histologic-radiologic correlations.[11] It is a 5-point ordinal scale:

1. Normal periapical structures
2. Small changes in bone structure with no dimineralization
3. Changes in bone structure with some diffuse demineralization
4. Apical periodontitis with well-defined radiolucent area
5. Severe apical periodontitis, with exacerbating features

The PAI, therefore, provides more objective criteria for radiographic evaluation of periapical status of teeth that have undergone endodontic treatment. Consequently, it has been used in several endodontic outcome studies for the assessment of periapical status.[12–15]

Recently, cone beam CT (CBCT) has found considerable applications in endodontic diagnosis and treatment planning.[16] The CBCT-PAI was developed to apply standardization in approaches to assess the severity of apical periodontitis by CBCT. This index is a 6-point scale that includes a score (0–5) plus 2 variables that assess expansion and destruction of cortical bone. The CBCT-PAI scale is as follows:

0: Intact periapical bone structures
1: Diameter of periapical radiolucency 0.5 mm to 1 mm
2: Diameter of periapical radiolucency 1 mm to 2 mm
3: Diameter of periapical radiolucency 2 mm to 4 mm
4: Diameter of periapical radiolucency 4 mm to 8 mm
5: Diameter of periapical radiolucency 8 mm
E: Expansion of periapical cortical bone
D: Destruction of periapical cortical bone

CBCT is more sensitive than conventional periapical radiography for detection of apical radiolucencies. Thus, it can be expected that the CBCT-PAI likely reduces the number of false-negative diagnoses on periapical radiographs. A recent study demonstrated, however, significant variation in the periodontal ligament space morphology of clinically healthy teeth.[17] This underscores the need to better evaluate and clearly define normal and abnormal features on CBCT imaging before considering systematic application of this new technology to outcomes assessment.

## INCONSISTENCY OF OUTCOME DEFINITIONS

Over the years, the terms, *success* and *failure*, came under close scrutiny due to discrepancies in clinical, histologic, and radiographic observations.[5] New modifiers and criteria were added, such as *stringent* and *lenient*,[18] and *strict* and *loose*.[19,20] This became confusing for practicing dentists who had to decipher the terminology and apply it to clinical assessment of endodontic outcome. Escalating the debate and controversy on endodontic treatment outcomes was the misleading comparison of endodontic treatment outcomes to the success rate of a single-tooth implant.[21,22] The term, *success*, was based on entirely different criteria for 2 treatment modalities.

A series of articles, now known as the Toronto Study,[13–15] introduced yet another set of terms deemed more appropriate to assess endodontic treatment results. The assessment of outcome was based on the PAI and categorized outcomes as "healed" when the PAI score is less than 3 or "disease" for PAI scores greater than or equal to 3. A novel category, "functional," was introduced for all teeth that were asymptomatic, regardless of PAI score. Subsequently, it was proposed that that endodontic treatment outcome should be expressed in terms of the healing of disease, and new terms, *healed, healing, disease,* and *functional retention,* were proposed.[22]

## THE AMERICAN ASSOCIATION OF ENDODONTISTS OUTCOME CRITERIA

With successful endodontic treatment, the periradicular inflammatory changes resolve and the osseous and periodontal structures regenerate around the tooth apex. For these changes to be radiographically apparent, there must adequate remineralization of the bone that may occur over an extended period of time. This emphasizes the need to consider the radiographic changes in the context of the tooth's functional status and clinical symptoms. Recognizing this, the AAE took the lead to review the existing criteria used in endodondontics and compared these to the outcome measures used by other specialties. The organization subsequently defined new terms for outcome assessment using valid measures that are appropriate for endodontics. As an alternative to the widely used Strindberg criteria, the new definitions were approved.[23]

## THE AMERICAN ASSOCIATION OF ENDODONTISTS–APPROVED DEFINITIONS OF ENDODONTIC OUTCOMES

- Healed — functional*, asymptomatic teeth with no or minimal radiographic periradicular pathosis (see **Figs. 1**C; **3**B; **4**C; **5**E, F; **7**E; and **8**D)
- Nonhealed — nonfunctional, symptomatic teeth with or without radiographic periradicular pathosis (see **Figs. 2**B, C; **5**C, D; **6**B–E; and **7**B, C)
- Healing — teeth with periradicular pathosis, which are asymptomatic and functional, or teeth with or without radiographic periradicular pathosis, which are symptomatic but whose intended function is not altered (see **Fig. 8**C)
- Functional* — a treated tooth or root that is serving its intended purpose in the dentition

## CONE BEAM COMPUTED TOMOGRAPHY–BASED OUTCOME ASSESSMENT

Over the past few years, CBCT has been used increasingly in endodontic diagnosis and treatment planning, with intent to incorporate this technology to better assess treatment decisions and outcomes.[24,25] The AAE and the American Academy of

Oral and Maxillofacial Radiology (AAOMR) jointly developed guidelines for the appropriate use of CBCT imaging in endodontics. These guidelines define clinical scenarios and 2-D radiographic appearances that are likely to benefit from CBCT imaging. CBCT is more sensitive than periapical radiography to detect bone lesions; thus, its use to evaluate outcomes will undoubtedly be beneficial to identify cases that would be false negatives on periapical radiography. Despite its higher accuracy for detecting

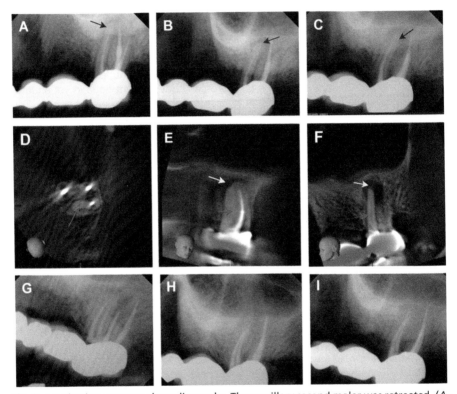

**Fig. 9.** Monitoring outcomes by radiography. The maxillary second molar was retreated. (A–C) Periapical radiographs taken at different horizontal angulations to evaluate endodontically treated symptomatic maxillary left second molar. Note the presence of a radiolucency around the mesiobuccal root apex (*blue arrow*). This represents a treatment failure according to Strindberg criteria and nonhealing according to the AAE classification. (D–F). Axial, coronal, and sagittal CBCT sections, respectively, through the maxillary second molar. Note the presence of an untreated second mesiobuccal canal (*red arrow*), that is not evident on the periapical radiographs. The extent of the lytic changes (*yellow arrows*) are better visualized on the CBCT sections, compared with the periapical radiographs. (G–I) Periapical radiographs made at completion of endodontic retreatment and 6-month and 30-month recall visits, respectively. The tooth continued to be clinically asymptomatic. The progressive resolution of apical periodontitis is consistent with a successful outcome (Strindberg criteria) and/or healed classification of outcome (AAE). Note that in the absence of symptoms, conventional imaging is adequate to document this successful outcome. Additional imaging with CBCT at these follow-up stages is unnecessary and unjustified. (*Courtesy of* Dr Nadia Chugal and Dr Sotirios Tetradis. *From* Chugal N, Mallya SM, Kahler B. Criteria for outcome assessment of non-surgical endodontic treatment. In: Chugal N, Lin LM, editors. Endodontic prognosis: clinical guide for optimal treatment outcome. 1st edition. Springer International Publishing Switzerland, 2017. With permission of Springer.)

periapical disease, the AAE-AAOMR guidelines recommend against using CBCT as a routine diagnostic and outcome assessment tool.[26]

The role of CBCT imaging in endodontics is illustrated by a case that highlights the value of CBCT as a powerful diagnostic tool that alters diagnosis and treatment plans (**Fig. 9**). The decision to proceed with CBCT was made only after clinical examination and 2-D radiography. Additional information provided by the CBCT examination was critical in elucidating the cause of endodontic failure by identifying an untreated infected canal. It is important for clinicians to recognize that CBCT imaging does not replace conventional imaging for documentation of case completion and outcome assessment. Whereas CBCT is of value in potentially identifying causes of endodontic treatment failure, the use of CBCT imaging only to monitor treatment outcome for asymptomatic teeth is unjustified.

## OUTCOME RATES FOR ORTHOGRADE ENDODONTIC TREATMENT

The results of Strindberg's seminal study[6] on outcomes of endodontic treatment at the end of the 4-year follow-up are presented (**Table 1**). These data demonstrate that success rates for endodontic treatment are significantly lower for necrotic teeth with apical periodontitis than for the teeth with a normal periapex ($P<.05$). The rates for aggregate analysis and stratification on preoperative periapical diagnosis demonstrate the intimate relationship between endodontic diagnosis and outcome of treatment. Therefore, the presence of a preoperative periapical radiolucency, denoting apical periodontitis, represents a powerful prognostic indicator.[6] This finding has been repeatedly demonstrated in several outcome studies that followed.[13,20,27–29] Studies on teeth with apical periodontitis that incorporated microbiologic sampling into the clinical protocol showed that teeth with positive culture prior to obturation had significantly lower rate of success compared with teeth that had negative culture results.[28,30,31] Similar findings have been demonstrated in studies using PAI score for measuring the healing.[13]

A systematic review of clinical studies pertaining to success and failure of nonsurgical endodontic treatment reported an overall radiographic success rate of 81.5% over a period of 5 years.[32] The wide range of reported success rates in individual studies was attributed to the criteria used.[19,20] Common to all these studies, however, is a significantly lower success rate for infected teeth with preoperative apical periodontitis.

**Table 1**
**Therapeutic results at 4-year and final follow-up examinations**

|  | Success (%) | Failure (%) | Uncertain (%) |
|---|---|---|---|
| No radiolucency | 89.16 | 8.04 | 2.80 |
| Yes radiolucency | 68.40 | 29.00 | 2.60 |
| Overall rate | 80.79 | 16.49 | 2.71 |

A significant difference exists in outcome rates between cases with preoperative periapical radiolucency compared with those with normal periapex ($P<.05$).[6]

## OUTCOME ASSESSMENT OF ENDODONTIC THERAPIES FOR IMMATURE TEETH

The primary goal of conventional endodontic treatment is prevention and/or elimination of apical periodontitis. The additional goals of endodontic treatment of immature teeth with an open apex are broader and include preservation of pulp vitality and promotion of root development to maturity or promotion of reparative processes when nascent physiologic mechanism is no longer possible due to pulp necrosis and apical periodontitis. To that end, there is an array of specific treatment protocols and options for young patients with developing dentition. Consequently, the outcome assessment of these therapies includes additional criteria to those outlined for mature teeth and their functional status[6,23] and are specific to the stage of root development and pulpal and periapical diagnosis.

### Vital Pulp Therapy

The overall goal of vital pulp therapy is to preserve vitality and functionality of dentin-pulp complex in a tooth that has been challenged with caries, iatrogenic pulp exposure or a traumatic injury, and diagnosed clinically with reversible pulpitis. The ultimate goal of the treatment is to promote growth and maturation of the immature root and thereby preserve the natural dentition in young patients. Current clinical protocols are based on the concept of up-regulation of functional activity of primary odontoblasts to produce reactionary dentinogenesis in indirect pulp capping,[33,34] and recruitment and differentiation of postnatal progenitor/stem cells in the uninfected vital pulp into secondary odontoblast-like cells to produce reparative dentinogenesis in direct pulp capping and pulpotomy.[34,35] Bioactive growth/differentiation factors embedded in the dentin matrix are capable of stimulating primary odontoblasts and progenitor/stem cells in the dental pulp to produce reactionary and reparative dentin, respectively.[34,35] A coordinated interplay between the Hertwig epithelial root sheath and apical papilla is required to promote apexogenesis.[36,37] Vital pulp therapy includes the following procedures.

### Indirect and direct pulp capping

Indirect pulp capping procedures do not involve direct manipulation of pulp tissue and preserve nascent odontoblasts, whereas direct pulp capping involves placement of dental material, such as calcium hydroxide, mineral trioxide aggregate (MTA,) or other bioceramic or calcium silicate–based cements directly over an exposed pulp but without pulp tissue removal.

### Pulpotomy

The pulpotomy procedure involves selective partial pulp amputation based on the extent of pulpal injury as assessed clinically. Inflamed pulp, either through caries process or trauma, is removed until hemostasis is attained and healthy-appearing pulp tissue is reached. The remaining pulp stump is covered with an appropriate dental material to promote hard tissue deposition and apexogenesis.

Many factors may affect the outcome of vital pulp therapy, such as age of patients, stage of tooth development, severity of pulp damage, regenerative potential of the pulp, and microleakage of the capping materials. Control of infection, however, seems to play the most important role in vital pulp therapy.[38]

## OUTCOME ASSESSMENT OF VITAL PULP THERAPY
### Success

Clinical
- Regression of clinical symptoms
- Maintenance of pulp vitality

Radiographic
- Progressive root growth in length (**Figs. 10** and **11**)
- Maturation of the apex (see **Figs. 10** and **11**)
- Thickening of the root canal walls (see **Figs. 10** and **11**)

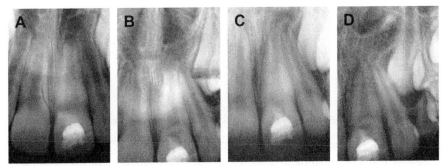

**Fig. 10.** Successful vital pulp therapy with calcium hydroxide of an immature tooth. Asymptomatic vital maxillary left central incisor tooth treated within 4 hours of injury. (*A*) Immediate postoperative periapical radiograph. (*B–D*) Periapical radiographs made at 6, 12, and 18 months after treatment showing completion of root development and apical closure by 18 months. Tooth remained asymptomatic, responsive to vitality tests and was functional. Incidental finding is calcific bridge formation at the level of cementoenamel junction. (*Courtesy of* N. Chugal, DDS, MS, MPH, Los Angeles, California.)

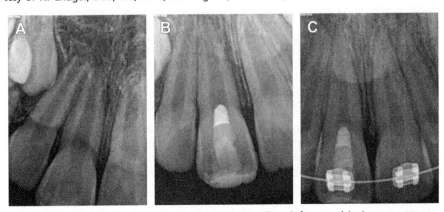

**Fig. 11.** Successful vital pulp therapy with MTA. Maxillary left central incisor was traumatized a year ago and was asymptomatic until 3 weeks ago. Although symptomatic, tooth exhibited normal response to pulp vitality tests. A deep pulpotomy with MTA was performed. (*A*) Preoperative periapical radiograph showing open root apices consistent with ongoing root development. Note absence of radiographic signs of apical periodontal inflammation. (*B*) Postoperative periapical radiograph demonstrating the extent of pulpotomy. (*C*) Periapical radiographs made 4 years after completion of treatment. Complete closure of root apices and establishment of normal periradicular structures demonstrate a successful outcome. Incidental finding is calcific bridge formation below MTA. (*Courtesy of* E.S. Perry, DMD, Westfield, Massachusetts.)

*Failure*

Clinical
- Persistence or recurrence of clinical symptoms
- Loss of pulp vitality

Radiographic
- Cessation of root growth (**Figs. 12** A–B)
- Cessation of maturation of the apex (**Figs. 12** A–B)
- Lack of thickening of root canal walls (**Figs. 12** A–B)

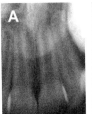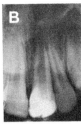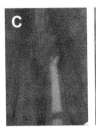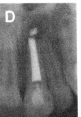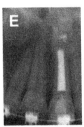

Fig. 12. Successful apexification with calcium hydroxide therapy. Traumatic injury to the maxillary left central incisor resulted in coronal fracture with pulp exposure. The tooth tested vital and direct pulp capping was performed. Eight months later, the tooth developed symptoms and was nonresponsive to pulp vitality tests. (A) Periapical radiograph taken at the time of traumatic injury showed an incompletely developed root of the left central incisor, with thin radicular walls and open apex. Trabecular bone around the apex is slightly radiolucent, indicative of periapical inflammation. (B) Follow-up radiography 8 months after trauma. Root development of the adjacent teeth is complete. Root formation of the maxillary left central incisor is arrested. Apexification therapy with calcium hydroxide was initiated. (C) Periapical radiograph taken after 6 months of apexification treatment and obturation with gutta percha. (D, E) Periapical radiographs made 12 and 24 months after apexification therapy completion and canal obturation. Note resolution of the periapical radiolucency and establishment of normal periodontal ligament and periradicular trabecular bone. This is also an example of unsuccessful vital pulp therapy and successful apexification. (Courtesy of N. Chugal, DDS, MS, MPH, Los Angeles, California.)

## OUTCOME RATES FOR VITAL PULP THERAPY

A systematic review of vital pulp therapy in permanent teeth with carious pulp exposure showed that the success rates after 3-year follow-up were 72.9% for direct pulp capping and up to 99.4% for pulpotomy.[39] Therefore, immature teeth seem to have better treatment outcomes than mature teeth presumably due to a greater immunologic and reparative response provided from an open apex.

### Apexification

Conventional root canal therapy for immature permanent teeth with a necrotic pulp is challenging because of thin, fragile canal walls, and divergent open apex. Therefore, when the pulps of immature permanent teeth become necrotic, traditionally, apexification is the treatment of choice. Apexification is defined as a method to induce a calcified barrier in a root with an open apex or the continued apical development of an incompletely formed root in teeth with necrotic pulps.[40] Apexification of immature permanent teeth with necrotic pulps can be achieved by calcium hydroxide dressing[41–43] or MTA[44,45] to create an apical barrier to prevent extrusion of root canal filling into the periapical tissues.

Calcium hydroxide apexification usually takes many months to induce apical hard tissue barrier and patient compliance may be problematic.[46] MTA apexification can be completed in 1 to 3 visits.[46] Consequently, MTA apexification has become the preferred treatment option.[46] The major drawback of apexification, however, is that the canal walls remain thin and are more prone to cervical root fracture.[47] The frequency of cervical root fracture ranges from 28% to 77% depending on the extent of the root development.[47] It has also been shown that a long-term calcium hydroxide dressing in the canal space of immature permanent teeth may weaken thin root structure, increasing the likelihood of root fractures.[48]

## OUTCOME ASSESSMENT OF APEXIFICATION PROCEDURES
### Success

Clinical
- Regression of clinical symptoms

Radiographic
- Resolution of apical radiolucency (**Figs. 12** and **13**)

### Failure

Clinical
- Persistence or recurrence of clinical symptoms

Radiographic
- Lack of resolution of periapical radiolucency
- Increased size of periapical radiolucency

## OUTCOME RATES FOR APEXIFICATION THERAPY

Apexification of immature teeth with necrotic pulps has been practiced for many decades with predictable high success rate in terms of elimination of clinical symptom/sign and radiographic resolution of periapical lesion.[46] According to a systematic review and meta-analysis comparing apexification of immature teeth with calcium hydroxide to that of MTA, the clinical outcome of the 2 treatments is similar in clinical success.[49] The most recent systematic review and meta-analysis comparing MTA and calcium hydroxide apexification of immature permanent teeth reported the clinical success rate range from 93% to 100% in the MTA groups and from 87% to 100% in the calcium hydroxide groups. The radiographic success rate was 100% in the MTA groups and ranged from 87% to 93% for the calcium hydroxide groups. Statistical analysis showed no significant difference in clinical and radiographic success between calcium hydroxide and MTA apexification.[50]

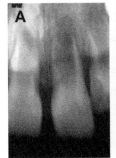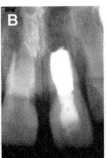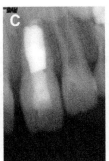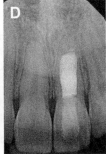

**Fig. 13.** Successful apexification with MTA therapy. (*A*) Periapical radiograph shows maxillary left central incisors with incomplete root development and open apices. Trabecular bone around the apex of the left central incisor is radiolucent suggestive of periradicular inflammation. Canal debridement was initiated and subsequently apexification therapy with MTA apical barrier completed, followed by canal obturation with gutta percha. (*B*) Follow-up radiography after 3 months. (*C, D*) Periapical radiograph taken 11 months and 8 years following apexification. Note resolution of the periapical radiolucency, root growth beyond apical extent of MTA, and establishment of normal periodontal ligament and periradicular trabecular bone around the apex of the left central incisor. Development of the right central incisor root is complete. (*Courtesy of* E.S. Perry, DMD, Westfield, Massachusetts.)

### Regenerative Endodontics

In 2001, a new treatment procedure, termed, *revascularization*, was introduced and involved an immature permanent tooth with a necrotic pulp and apical periodontitis.[51] This case report described a technique that allowed further root maturation with thickening of the canal walls and apical closure. Therefore, the major limitation of the traditional apexification where the root walls remain thin could be overcome with the potential for strengthening of the root with apposition of new mineralized tissue with this biologically based treatment. Since then, there have been many published reports attesting to the efficacy of regenerative endodontic protocols, which generally involve a 2-visit procedure.[52] The AAE guidelines recommend that the first visit involve disinfection of the root canal space with 1.5% sodium hypochlorite and placement of an intracanal antimicrobial dressing of either a triple antibiotic paste composed of minocycline, ciprofloxacin, and metronidazole or calcium hydroxide. At a second appointment, the medicament is irrigated with 17% EDTA.[53] EDTA releases growth factors from the dentin matrix and exposes specific binding sites in the root dentin.[54] The periapical tissues are then lacerated to induce bleeding into the canal and blood clot formation, just below the cementoenamel junction. Stem cells from the apical papilla and progenitor cells are introduced in the canal to facilitate further root maturation. An intracanal barrier of MTA is placed over the blood clot and the access cavity is restored with glass ionomer cement and composite resin.[53] There have been many variations in the materials used for this technique with no standardized protocol.[55]

Several different terms have used to describe this procedure, including revascularization and revitalization, although the term, *regenerative endodontics*, has become more acceptable.[52] Histologic studies have shown, however, that the newly derived tissue is not pulplike and is derived from the periodontium with cementum, osteoidlike, and connective tissue found in the canal.[56,57] Therefore, the regenerative endodontic technique seems to promote repair rather than true regeneration. It is hoped that with refinements to the protocol and the inclusion of bioengineering approaches, such as scaffolds, bioactive growth factors, and chemoattractants, that true regeneration of the pulp can be attained.[58]

## OUTCOME ASSESSMENT OF REGENERATIVE ENDODONTIC PROCEDURES

The degree of success of regenerative endodontic procedures (REPs) is largely measured by the extent to which it is possible to attain primary, secondary, and tertiary goals.[59] Accordingly, current guidelines by the AAE[53] define success of REPs by these 3 measures:

1. Primary goal (essential): the elimination of symptoms and the evidence of bony healing
2. Secondary goal (desirable): increased root wall thickness and/or increased root length
3. Tertiary goal: positive response to vitality testing

In addition, tooth discoloration is an adverse risk of the procedure and should be considered a patient-centered outcome.[60]

The AAE recommendations for evaluation at follow-up clinical and radiographic examinations are listed[53] and are presented in a format that parallels those of other orthograde endodontic procedures for mature teeth[6,23]:

### Success

Clinical
- No pain, soft tissue swelling, or sinus tract (often observed between first and second appointments) (primary goal)
- Response to pulp vitality tests (tertiary goal)

Radiographic
- Resolution of apical radiolucency (often observed 6–12 months after treatment) (primary goal) (**Figs. 14–17**)
- Increased width of root walls (this is generally observed before apparent increase in root length and often occurs 12–24 months after treatment) (secondary goal) (see **Figs. 14–17**)
- Increased root length (secondary goal) (see **Fig. 17**)

*Failure*

- Nonattainment of primary goal

## OUTCOME RATES FOR REGENERATIVE ENDODONTIC THERAPY

Studies to date report that healing of apical periodontitis occurred in greater than 90% of cases but changes in the extent of further root development were much more variable.[61] There are few systematic reviews of outcomes for REPs. Large clinical trials and prospective studies are needed to determine outcomes for teeth treated with REPs. Four cohort studies (level of evidence 2), however, have assessed changes in root width and length and all 4 reported that immature teeth treated with REPs showed increased root width and length.[62–65] All 4 studies also compared outcomes of REPs with traditional apexification with either calcium hydroxide and/or MTA and showed superior outcomes for teeth treated with REPs. Therefore, some investigators suggest that REPs may be considered the first treatment option for immature teeth with pulpal necrosis.[61]

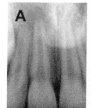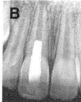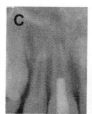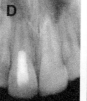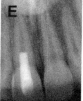

**Fig. 14.** Successful regenerative endodontic treatment. The maxillary right central incisor was painful on presentation and recently exhibited discoloration of the crown. The tooth sustained trauma approximately 6 months ago and tested nonvital indicating pulpal necrosis. (*A*) Periapical radiograph shows the apex of the maxillary right central incisor with an open root apex and a periapical radiolucency, consistent with the clinical manifestations of pulpal necrosis. (*B*) Postoperative radiograph of tooth treated with REPs. (*C*) Periapical radiograph showing partial resolution of the periapical radiolucency around the right central incisor, consistent with resolution of clinical symptoms. Overall, the appearance is indicative of healing of the periapical inflammation. (*D*) Periapical radiograph showing resolution of the periapical radiolucency with evidence of osseous healing and re-establishment of the periodontal ligament space and lamina dura around the apex of the right central incisor. Note minimal changes in the width of the apical foramen. (*E*) Follow-up radiography after 4 years confirms closure of root apex, with no periapical rarefaction, confirming successful regenerative endodontic treatment. There is thickening of the root wall apical to MTA that was placed into the coronal one-third of the canal. Incidental finding: dispersed throughout apical two-thirds of the canal are radiopacities suggesting ectopic calcifications. (*Courtesy of* E.S. Perry, DMD, Westfield, Massachusetts.)

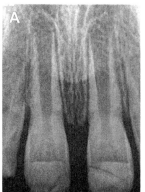
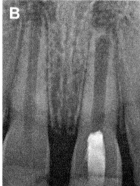
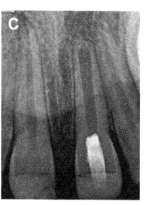

**Fig. 15.** Successful regenerative endodontic treatment. Maxillary central incisors sustained an uncomplicated crown fracture and were initially treated with composite resin. After 6 months, the patient presented with pain and swelling of the maxillary left central incisor and was treated with REPs. (*A*) Periapical radiograph taken at the time of trauma demonstrating incomplete root development of the maxillary incisors. (*B*) Postoperative radiograph after REPs after maxillary left central incisor became symptomatic. MTA was placed over the blood clot at the level of cementoenamel junction. Note perceptible decrease in the size of the apical foramen relative to the pretreatment radiograph, suggesting necrosis did not develop immediately after trauma. (*C*) Periapical radiograph taken 18 months after regenerative treatment, showing evident decrease in the size of the apical foramen, with closure of the root apex. Note that the development of the apex of the left central incisor is delayed, relative to the right central incisor. There is no additional increase in root length compared with the right central incisor and radicular dentin deposition is occurring at a slower rate. There is closure, however, of the apex and the reestablishment of the periapical structures. (*Courtesy of* E.S. Perry, DMD, Westfield, Massachusetts.)

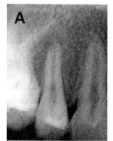
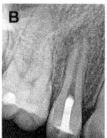
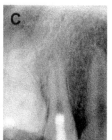
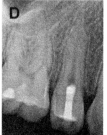

**Fig. 16.** Successful regenerative endodontic treatment. (*A*) Pretreatment periapical radiograph demonstrating a diffuse radiolucency around the apex of incompletely formed apex of the second premolar. (*B*) Postoperative radiograph made after canal disinfection and subsequent regenerative endodontic treatment. MTA was placed at the level of cementoenamel junction. (*C*) Periapical radiograph taken 9 months after regenerative treatment. Note resolution of the periapical radiolucency, with minimal but perceptible decrease in the width of the apical canal. (*D*) Periapical radiograph taken 18 months after regenerative treatment. Note complete closure of the apex and the re-establishment of the periodontal ligament space and the lamina dura. There seems to be minimal increase in canal wall thickness but significant intracanal calcification of the apical third of root. (*Courtesy of* E.S. Perry, DMD, Westfield, Massachusetts.)

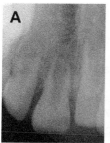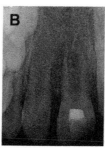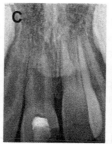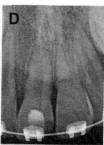

**Fig. 17.** Successful regenerative endodontic treatment. (*A*) Pretreatment periapical radiograph shows a radiolucency around the apex of the maxillary right central incisor and incomplete root development. (*B*) Postoperative radiograph after REPs. Note MTA placement above the cementoenamel junction. (*C*) Periapical radiograph taken 15 months after REPs. The periapical radiolucency is resolved. The width of the apical pulp canal is narrowed, but the apex is not completely closed. The root length is slightly shorter relative to the left central incisor, suggestive of arrested root growth in length. (*D*) Periapical radiograph taken 27 months after REPs. Calcification of the apical portion of the canal, with closure of the root and formation of the apical periodontal ligament space and periradicular trabecular bone is evident. Incidental finding is radiopacities at the apical extent of the canal and at the level of cementoenamel junction, which may represent dentinal/calcific bridge formation. Teeth #7 and #10 exhibit normal growth and development. Tooth #9 underwent calcific metamorphosis. (*Courtesy of* E.S. Perry, DMD, Westfield, Massachusetts.)

## SUMMARY

Assessment of endodontic treatment outcomes has evolved from disease-based criteria proposed by Strindberg to patient-centered values, emphasizing survival and function of endodontically treated teeth even in the presence of inflammatory periapical disease. It is important that patients are fully informed of the difference between disease-free and disease-associated treatment outcome. Ideally, disease-free treatment outcome should always be the goal of all endodontic treatments.

## ACKNOWLEDGMENTS

We wish to express our deep appreciation for the meticulously documented clinical cases and radiographic images provided by our colleagues, Dr Charles Maupin, Dr David Han, Dr Alexis Moore, and Dr. Elizabeth Shin Perry, who are referenced in the figure legends. These images provided excellent illustrations for the concepts presented and we thank them for their contributions.

## REFERENCES

1. Pak JG, White SN. Pain prevalence and severity before, during, and after root canal treatment: a systematic review. J Endod 2011;37:429–38.
2. Nixdorf DR, Moana-Filho EJ, Law AS, et al. Frequency of persistent tooth pain after root canal therapy: a systematic review and meta-analysis. J Endod 2010;36:224–30.
3. Lin L, Pascon E, Skirbner J, et al. Clinical, radiographic, and histologic study of endodontic treatment failures. Oral Surg Oral Med Oral Pathol 1991;71:603–11.
4. Bender IB, Seltzer S, Soltanoff W. Endodontic success–a reappraisal of criteria. 1. Oral Surg Oral Med Oral Pathol 1966;22:780–9.

5. Bender IB, Seltzer S, Soltanoff W. Endodontic success-a reappraisal of criteria. II. Oral Surg Oral Med Oral Pathol 1966;22:790–802.
6. Strindberg LZ. The dependence of the results of pulp therapy on certain factors. Acta Odontol Scand 1956;14:1–175.
7. Bender IB, Seltzer S. Roentgenographic and direct observation of experimental lesions in bone: part I. J Am Dent Assoc 1961;62:152–60.
8. Goldman M, Pearson AH, Darzenta N. Endodontic success-who's reading the radiograph? Oral Surg Oral Med Oral Pathol 1972;33:432–7.
9. Gelfand M, Sunderman EJ, Goldman M. Reliability of radiographical interpretations. J Endod 1983;9:71–5.
10. Ørstavik D, Kerekes K, Eriksen HM. The periapical index: a scoring system for radiographic assessment of apical periodontitis. Endod Dent Traumatol 1986;2: 20–34.
11. Brynolf I. A histologic and roentgenologic study of the periapical region of human upper incisors. Odontol Revy Suppl 1967;11:1–176.
12. Ørstavik D, Kerekes K, Eriksen HM. Clinical performance of three endodontic sealers. Endod Dent Traumatol 1987;3:178–86.
13. Friedman S, Abitbol S, Lawrence HP. Treatment outcome in endodontics: the Toronto Study. Phase 1: initial treatment. J Endod 2003;29:787–93.
14. Farzaneh M, Abitbol S, Lawrence HP, et al, Toronto Study. Treatment outcome in endodontics-the Toronto Study. Phase II: initial treatment. J Endod 2004;30:302–9.
15. de Chevigny C, Dao TT, Basrani BR, et al. Treatment outcome in endodontics: the Toronto study–phase 4: initial treatment. J Endod 2008;34:258–63.
16. Estrela C, Bueno MR, Azevedo BC, et al. A new periapical index based on cone beam computed tomography. J Endod 2008;34:1325–31.
17. Pope O, Sathorn C, Parashos P. A comparative investigation of cone-beam computed tomography and periapical radiography in the diagnosis of a healthy periapex. J Endod 2014;40:360–5.
18. Friedman S. Prognosis of initial endodontic therapy. Endod Top 2002;2:59–88.
19. Ng YL, Mann V, Rahbaran S, et al. Outcome of primary root canal treatment: systematic review of the literature - part 1. Effects of study characteristics on probability of success. Int Endod J 2007;40:921–39.
20. Ng YL, Mann V, Gulabivala K. A prospective study of the factors affecting outcomes of non-surgical root canal treatment: part 2: tooth survival. Int Endod J 2011;44:610–25.
21. Albrektsson T, Zarb G, Worthington P, et al. The long-term efficacy of currently used dental implants: a review and proposed criteria of success. Int J Oral Maxillofac Implants 1986;1:11–25.
22. Friedman S, Mor C. The success of endodontic therapy-healing and functionality. J Calif Dent Assoc 2004;32:493–503.
23. The American Association of Endodontists Communiqué. AAE and Foundation approve definition of Endodontic Outcomes. Volume XXIX, August/September 2005. Page 3.
24. Wu MK, Shemesh H, Wesselink PR. Limitations of previously published systematic reviews evaluating the outcome of endodontic treatment. Int Endod J 2009;42:656–66.
25. Patel S, Mannocci F, Shemesh H, et al. Editorial. Int Endod J 2011;44:887–8.
26. American Association of Endodontists and American Academy of Oral and Maxillofacial Radiology Position Statement. 2015. Available at: http://c.ymcdn.com/sites/www.aaomr.org/resource/resmgr/Docs/AAOMR-AAE_postition_paper_CB.pdf. Accessed September 03, 2016.

27. Kerekes K, Tronstad L. Long-term results of endodontic treatment performed with a standardized technique. J Endod 1979;5:83–90.
28. Sjögren U, Hågglund B, Sundqvist G, et al. Factors affecting the long-term results of endodontic treatment. J Endod 1990;16:498–504.
29. Chugal NM, Clive JM, Spångberg LSW. A prognostic model for assessment of the outcome of endodontic treatment: effect of biologic and diagnostic variables. Oral Surg Oral Med Oral Pathol Oral Radiol Endod 2001;91:342–52.
30. Engström B, Segerstad LHA, Ramström G, et al. Correlation of positive cultures with the prognosis for root canal treatment. Odontol Revy 1964;15:257–70.
31. Sjögren U, Figdor D, Persson S, et al. Influence of infection at the time of root filling on the outcome of endodontic treatment of teeth with apical periodontitis. Int Endod J 1997;30:297–306.
32. Torabinejad M, Kutsenko D, Machnick TK, et al. Levels of evidence for the outcome of nonsurgical endodontic treatment. J Endod 2005;31:637–46.
33. Smith AJ, Tobias N, Perry H, et al. Reactionary dentinogenesis. Int J Dev Biol 1995;39:273–80.
34. Tziafas D. The future role of a molecular approach to pulp-dentin regeneration. Caries Res 2004;38:314–20.
35. Smith AJ. Dentin formation and repair. In: Hargreaves KM, Goodis HE, Tay FR, et al, editors. Dental pulp. Chicago: Quintessence; 2012.
36. Sonoyama W, Liu Y, Yamaza T, et al. Characterization of the apical papilla and its residing stem cells from human immature permanent teeth: a pilot study. J Endod 2008;34:166–71.
37. Zeichner-David M, Oishi K, Su Z, et al. Role of Hertwig's epithelial root sheath cells in tooth root development. Dev Dyn 2003;228:651–63.
38. Ricucci D, Loghin S, Siqueira JF Jr. Correlation between clinical and histologic pulp diagnosis. J Endod 2014;40:1932–9.
39. Arguilar P, Linsuwanont P. Vital pulp therapy in vital permanent teeth with cariously exposed pulp: a systematic review. J Endod 2011;37:581–7.
40. American Association of Endodontists. Glossary of endodontic terms. 8th edition. Chicago: American Association of Endodontists; 2012.
41. Frank AL. Therapy for the divergent pulpless tooth by continued apical formation. J Am Dent Assoc 1966;72:87–93.
42. Cvek M. Treatment of non-vital permanent incisors with calcium hydroxide. I. Follow-up of periapical repair and apical closure of immature roots. Odonotol Revy 1972;23:27–44.
43. Heithersay GS. Calcium hydroxide in the treatment of pulpless teeth with associated pathology. J Br Endod Soc 1975;8:74–93.
44. Torabinejad M, Chivian N. Clinical applications of mineral trioxide aggregate. J Endod 1999;25:197–205.
45. Witherspoon DE, Ham K. One-visit apexification: technique for inducing root end barrier formation in apical closures. Pract Proced Aesthet Dent 2001;13:455–60.
46. Rafter M. Apexification: a review. Dent Traumatol 2005;21:1–8.
47. Cvek M. Prognosis of luxated non-vital maxillary incisors reated with calcium hydroxide and filled with gutta-percha, a retrospective clinical study. Endod Dent Traumatol 1992;8:45–55.
48. Andreasen JO, Farik B, Munksgaard EC. Long-term calcium hydroxide as a root canal dressing may increase risk of root fracture. Dent Traumatol 2002;18:134–7.
49. Chala S, Abouqal R, Rida S, et al. Apexification with calcium hydroxide or mineral trioxide aggregate: systematic review and meta-analysis. Oral Surg Oral Med Oral Pathol Oral Radiol Endod 2011;112:36–42.

50. Lin JC, Lu JX, Zeng O, et al. Comparison of mineral trioxide aggregate and calcium hydroxide for apexification of immature permanent teeth: a systematic review and meta-analysis. J Formos Med Assoc 2016;115:523–30.
51. Iwaya S, Ikawa M, Kubota M. Revascularization of an immature permanent tooth with apical periodontitis and sinus tract. Dent Traumatol 2001;17:185–7.
52. Diogenes A, Henry MA, Teixeira FB, et al. An update on clinical regenerative endodontics. Endod Top 2013;28:2–23.
53. American Association of Endodontists. AAE clinical considerations for a regenerative procedure. Available at: https://www.aae.org/uploadedfiles/publications_and_research/research/currentregenerativeendodonticconsiderations.pdf. Accessed September 03, 2016.
54. Galler KM, Buchalla W, Hiller KA, et al. Influence of root canal disinfectants on growth factor release from dentin. J Endod 2015;41:363–8.
55. Kontakiotis EG, Filippatos CG, Tzanetakis GN, et al. Regenerative endodontic therapy: a data analysis of clinical protocols. J Endod 2015;41:146–54.
56. Wang X, Thibodeau B, Trope M, et al. Histological characterization of regenerated tissues in canal space after revitalization/revascularization procedure of immature dog teeth with apical periodontitis. J Endod 2010;36:56–63.
57. Martin DE, De Almeida JF, Henry MA, et al. Concentration-dependent effect of sodium hypochlorite on stem cells of apical papilla survival and differentiation. J Endod 2014;40:51–5.
58. Hargreaves KM, Diogenes A, Teixeira FB. Paradigm lost: a perspective on the design and interpretation of regenerative endodontic research. J Endod 2014; 40:S65–9.
59. Geisler TM. Clinical considerations for regenerative endodontic procedures. Dent Clin North Am 2012;56:603–26.
60. Kahler B, Rossi-Fedele G. A review of tooth discoloration after regenerative endodontic therapy. J Endod 2016;42:563–9.
61. Diogenes A, Ruparel NB, Shiloah Y, et al. Regenerative endodontics. A way forward. J Am Dent Assoc 2016;147:372–80.
62. Bose R, Nummikoski P, Hargreaves K. A retrospective evaluation of radiographic outcomes in immature teeth with necrotic root canal systems treated with regenerative endodontic procedures. J Endod 2009;35:1343–9.
63. Jeeruphan T, Jantarat J, Yanpiset K, et al. Mahidol study 1: comparison of radiographic and survival outcomes of immature teeth treated with either regenerative endodontic or apexification methods—a retrospective study. J Endod 2012;38: 1330–6.
64. Nagy MM, Tawfik HE, Hashem AA, et al. Regenerative potential of immature permanent teeth with necrotic pulps after different regenerative protocols. J Endod 2014;40:192–8.
65. Alobaid AS, Cortes LM, Lo J, et al. Radiographic and clinical outcomes of the treatment of immature permanent teeth by revascularization or apexification: a pilot retrospective cohort study. J Endod 2014;40:1063–70.

# Modern Endodontic Microsurgery Concepts
## A Clinical Update

Spyros Floratos, DMD*, Syngcuk Kim, DDS, PhD

## KEYWORDS

- Microsurgery • Magnification • Surgical operating microscope • Isthmus
- Inspection • Apical surgery

## KEY POINTS

- Microsurgical technique is a minimally invasive procedure that results in faster healing and a better patient response.
- Inspection is the key stage of microsurgery that is completely missing from the older surgical technique.
- Untreated isthmuses frequently cause treatments to fail; therefore, they must be identified, cleaned, shaped, and filled as carefully as the root canals.
- By following a strict microsurgical protocol and careful patient selection, almost all lesions of endodontic origin can be successfully treated.

## ENDODONTIC MICROSURGERY: PROCEDURAL STEPS
### Flap Design

Semilunar incision was the most commonly used incision design in older surgical procedures, especially in the maxillary anterior area. This incision is no longer used, as it does not allow for an adequate access to the surgical site and is related to prolonged inflammation and scar formation on healing of the wound.[1] Modern microsurgery is using the triangular flap with 1 vertical incision, the papilla base incision for preservation of the papillae and the Lüebke-Ochsenbein submarginal flap. The last one is the most commonly used esthetic flap design especially in the maxillary anterior area. It is performed within the zone of the attached gingiva and results in almost zero recession of the gum margins and the interdental papillae postoperatively.[2,3] Therefore, crown margin exposure and formation of "black triangles" in anterior teeth as well as food impaction in posterior teeth is prevented. In microsurgical technique, vertical incisions should be 1.5 to 2 times longer

The authors have no conflict of interest to disclose.
Department of Endodontics, University of Pennsylvania School of Dental Medicine, 240S 40th Street, Philadelphia, PA 19104, USA
* Corresponding author. Private Practice, 13 Koniari Street, Athens 11471, Greece.
*E-mail address:* sflo_@hotmail.com

than in the traditional technique, so the flap is reflected far away from the light path of the microscope and adequate visibility of the surgical site is achieved.[4]

### Osteotomy

In microsurgery, osteotomy becomes more and more conservative thanks to the enhanced magnification and illumination offered by the microscope. The diameter of the osteotomy is only 3 to 4 mm, just enough to allow for a 3-mm ultrasonic tip to vibrate freely within the bone cavity (**Figs. 1** and **5**).[5] To prepare a small-size osteotomy, the exact position of the root apex has to be identified. The clinician has to have in mind the following guidelines:

- Sometimes the cortical plate is perforated and the perforation can be identified with a microexplorer under the microscope. In that case, the osteotomy site is obvious. A microexplorer also can penetrate through a thin layer of cortical bone underneath which lies the lesion.
- If there is a sound cortical bone, the measurement of the tooth length by using digital radiograph or even better by using cone-beam computed tomography (CBCT) can give us a precise estimation of the root apex position.
- If there is a periapical lesion extending on both roots of a lower molar, then starting the osteotomy right at the center of the lesion will safely lead us to both mesial and distal root apex.
- If the osteotomy does not reveal the root apex at a depth of 2 to 3 mm, the placement of a radiopaque material on the cortical bone, for example, gutta percha, resilon, aluminum foil, and the acquisition of a periapical radiograph is a clinical technique for root apex identification.

A small-size osteotomy leads to reduced postoperative discomfort and faster healing. A clinical study on healing, as evidenced by radiographic changes, showed that there is a

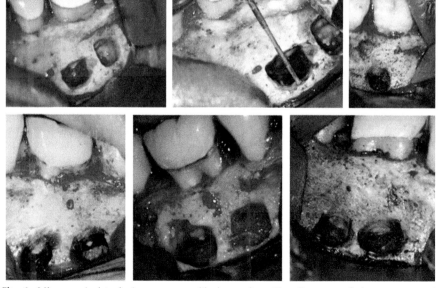

**Fig. 1.** Microsurgical technique on mandibular molars. The diameter of the osteotomy is only 3 to 4 mm, just enough to allow for a 3-mm ultrasonic tip to vibrate freely within the bone cavity. The root is resected at a 0° to 10° bevel.

direct relationship between the size of the osteotomy and the speed of healing: the smaller the osteotomy, the faster the healing. For instance, a lesion smaller than 5 mm would take an average of 6.4 months, a 6-mm to 10-mm-size lesion takes 7.25 months, and larger than 10 mm requires 11 months to heal.[6] Thus, the osteotomy should be as small as possible, but as large as necessary to accomplish the clinical objective.

## Root Resection

After granulation tissue is removed to the extent where the root apex is clearly visible, 3 mm of the root tip is resected perpendicular to the long axis of the root (**Fig. 4D**). A Lindemann bur should be used in any 45° angled handpiece using copious water spray. Some clinical guidelines during root resection are the following:

- 3 mm of root resection equals to approximately twice the width of a Lindemann bur.
- After resecting the root end, complete removal of all granulation tissue is facilitated, as there is often remaining granulation tissue behind the root tip.

Endodontic literature over the past 2 decades supports several reasons for resection of the apical part of the root during periapical surgery:

- Removal of pathologic processes.
- Removal of anatomic variations (apical deltas, accessory canals, apical ramifications, severe curves).
- Removal of iatrogenic mishaps (ledges, blockages, perforations, strip perforations, separated instruments).
- Enhanced removal of the granulation tissue.
- Access to the canal system when the coronal access is blocked or when coronal access with nonsurgical retreatment is determined to be impractical, time-consuming, and too invasive.
- Evaluation of the apical seal.
- Creation of an apical seal.
- Reduction of fenestrated root apices.
- Evaluation for complete or incomplete vertical root fractures.

There is no consensus concerning the amount of root that has to be resected. An anatomic study of the root apex conducted at the University of Pennsylvania revealed that at least 3 mm of the root end must be removed to reduce 98% of the apical ramifications and 93% of the lateral canals.[5]

To verify a complete resection of the root tip, the root surface has to be stained with methylene blue and inspected under a medium magnification ($\times 10-\times 12$) for the presence of the periodontal ligament (PDL).[7,8] When a complete root-end resection has been done, the PDL appears as an uninterrupted circular line around the root surface (**Fig. 2**). Incomplete root resection is one of the most common reasons for failure of a surgery.

## Root-End Resection: Long Bevel Versus Short Bevel

With traditional surgical technique, it was recommended that the angle of root-end resection should be 45° to 60° from the long axis of the root facing toward the buccal or facial aspect of the root.[9–12] However, there is no biological justification for creating a steep bevel on the resected root end. The steeper the bevel, the more potential for one of the following complications to occur[5,8,13]:

- Damage to or unnecessary removal of buccal supporting bone.

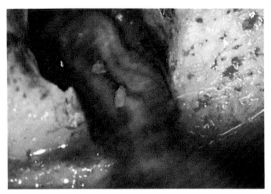

**Fig. 2.** Tooth #19 apical surgery. The resected surface on the mesial root is stained with methylene blue and inspected under a medium magnification (×12) for the presence of the PDL. When a complete root-end resection has been done, the PDL appears as an uninterrupted circular line around the root surface. Inspection also reveals the isthmus that joins the mesiobuccal and mesiolingual canal.

- Incomplete root resection: This can occur particularly on roots that extend rather deep lingually, such as the roots of a mandibular molar.
- Root canal anatomy missed on the lingual/palatal aspect of the root.

The operator's spatial disorientation regarding the true long axis of the canal system can be a result of the long bevel. This increases the risk of perforations of the lingual or palatal dentinal walls during root-end preparation (see section on root-end preparation). On the contrary, microsurgery suggests a 0° bevel, perpendicular to the long axis of the tooth (see **Fig. 1**).

*Inspection* under high magnification is the key stage of microsurgery that is missing from the traditional surgical technique.[5] A careful inspection will identify the possible reason or reasons for failure of the nonsurgical treatment. Inspection uses the high magnification and illumination that the operating microscope offers.[5–8,13,14] Magnification of the microscope should be set at the range of ×14 to ×25, higher than the rest of the surgical steps. During inspection, the resected root end is rinsed and dried with a Stropko Irrigator (Vista Dental, Racine, WI) (**Fig. 3**).

The dried surface is then stained with 1% methylene blue, which is applied to the root surface with a microapplicator tip.

Following that, a micromirror is placed at 45° to the resected surface and the reflected view of the root surface shows every anatomic detail of the canal system (**Fig. 4**A, B, and D).

The most common microfinding seen on inspection is a gap in the filling. That is essentially a space (stained with methylene blue) between the root canal filling material and the adjacent dentinal wall (**Fig. 4**C).

A complete evaluation involves not only the inspection of the cut root surface, but also of the whole root surface, particularly in cases in which there is a persistent lateral periradicular lesion evident on the radiograph or a lesion that extends alongside the entire length of the root. In this way, a vertical fracture, a perforation, or a lateral exit of an accessory canal may be found.

### Clinical Significance and Management of Isthmus

An isthmus is a narrow, ribbon-shaped communication between 2 root canals that contains pulp, or pulpally derived tissue (see **Fig. 2**; **Fig. 5**).[15] The isthmus is a part

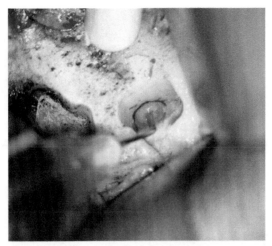

**Fig. 3.** Tooth #19 apical surgery. The resected surface on the distal root is stained with methylene blue and inspected under a medium magnification (×12). During inspection, the resected root end is dried with a Stropko Irrigator.

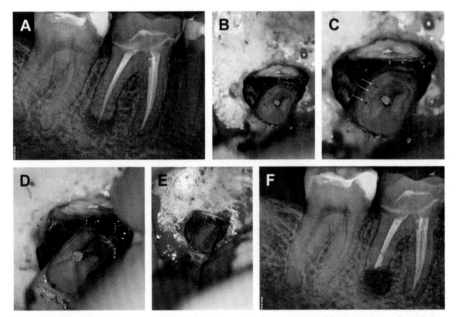

**Fig. 4.** (*A*) Failed previous endodontic treatment with a periapical lesion on tooth #30. Preoperative radiograph. Apical surgery by use of the microsurgical technique was determined. (*B*) Inspection of the resected root surface on the distal root was performed by placing a micromirror at a 45° angle to the resected surface (magnification ×8). (*C*) Inspection revealed a gap in the filling on the distal canal and 3 accessory canals (*white arrows*) (magnification ×12). (*D*) By resecting the root face 0.5 mm more coronally, the accessory canals were eliminated (magnification ×12). (*E*) Root-end filling with MTA on the distal canal (magnification ×12). (*F*) Postoperative radiograph showing a 3-mm root-end filling coaxial to the distal canal.

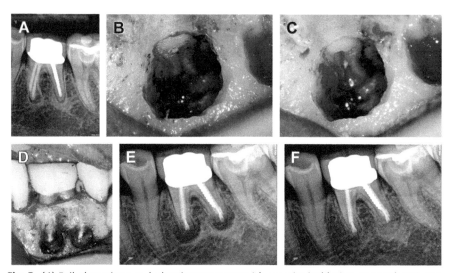

**Fig. 5.** (*A*) Failed previous endodontic treatment with a periapical lesion on tooth #19. Preoperative radiograph. Apical surgery by use of the microsurgical technique was determined. (*B*) Inspection of the resected root surface on the mesial root reveals an unprepared isthmus in between the 2 mesial canals (direct view-magnification ×12). (*C*) Root-end preparation on the mesial root by use of ultrasonics (direct view-magnification ×12). (*D*) Postoperative clinical view showing the small-size osteotomies and the root-end filling with bioceramic (Endosequence BC Root Repair Material, putty; Brasseler) on both roots (magnification ×8). (*E*) Postoperative radiograph showing a 3-mm root-end filling coaxial to the canals. (*F*) Radiographic examination at 12-month follow-up revealed complete bone healing.

of the canal system and not a separate entity. Therefore, it must be cleaned, shaped, and filled as thoroughly as possible. When performing apical surgery, the clinician should be aware that isthmuses are present in premolars and molars in approximately 80% to 90% of cases at the 3 mm level from the apex.[5,15,16]

When the apical segments of mesial roots of mandibular molars after apical surgery were examined under transmission electron microscopy, in 10 of the 11 root tips that had an isthmus, there were microorganisms present within the isthmus area. These findings prove that the isthmus tissue appears to be the "Achilles' heel" of conventional endodontic treatment.[17] Moreover, this is one of the reasons why apical root resection alone, without root-end preparation and root-end filling of canals and the isthmus, usually fails. Identification of unnegotiated canals and isthmuses is the first and most important step after root-end resection.

It is essential that the entire canal and isthmus be prepared to a depth of 3 mm. Clinical experience has shown that the main cause of failure after surgery in maxillary and mandibular premolars, mesiobuccal roots of maxillary molars, and mesial roots of mandibular molars, done with a bur and amalgam is the inability to treat the isthmus.[5,16,18]

### Root-End Preparation

Root-end preparation aims at removing the filling material, irritants, necrotic tissue, and remnants from the canals as well as the isthmus and creates a cavity that can be properly filled. The ideal root-end preparation is a class I cavity at least 3 mm into root dentin (**Fig. 4**F), with walls parallel to and within the anatomic outline of the root canal space (see **Fig. 5**).[19] This clinical demand can no longer be satisfied by use of rotary burs in a micro-handpiece, which was the common practice in traditional surgical techniques.

What is clinically important for an efficient ultrasonic preparation is not the brand or type of tip, but how the tip is used. In terms of pressure during ultrasonic preparation, the key is an extremely light touch in a repeated fashion. A lighter touch increases the cutting efficiency, whereas a continuous pressure, similar to the way a handpiece is used, decreases the cutting efficiency. That is because ultrasonics work through vibration, not through pressure. If resistance is met during ultrasonication, then a typical high-pitch sound is produced, indicating that the tip is cutting against dentin. At that point, the operator should stop the preparation, go to a low-range magnification of the microscope, realign the tip with the long axis of the root, and start again. If this step is not taken, then transportation or a perforation of the root might occur either on the lingual or distal dentinal wall.

The clinician should be aware of the following clinical concepts during root-end preparation:

- Root-end preparation begins with aligning a selected ultrasonic tip along the root prominence on the buccal plate under low magnification.
- ($\times$4–$\times$8) to ensure that the preparation follows the long axis of the root.
- Once the ultrasonic tip is aligned, the preparation is carried out under midrange magnification ($\times$10–$\times$12).
- Ultrasonic tips are used in a light, sweeping motion: short forward/backward and upward/downward strokes result in effective cutting action.
- Interrupted strokes are more effective than a continuous pressure on the dentin surface.

Once the apical preparation has been completed, gutta percha should be compacted with a microcondenser and the preparation should be dried and inspected with a micromirror. There should be a dry and clean class I cavity coaxial to the root, with no debris or tissue remnants and no filling material left on the axial walls (**Fig. 6**). Modern ultrasonic tips can facilitate the preparation of a 4-mm, 5-mm, 6-mm, or even 9-mm root-end cavity depending on the length of the unprepared canal space.

### *Root-End Filling*

Root-end filling is the last part of the surgical procedure and adequate hemostasis in the bone crypt as well as dryness in the root-end cavity is extremely important. For this reason, an epinephrine-impregnated cotton pellet is left at the depth of the osteotomy to maintain hemostasis as well as to prevent particles of the root-end filling material from falling at the periradicular bone or PDL.

Various materials have been used as root-end filling materials over the past few years: amalgam, gold foil, zinc oxide eugenol cements, Diaket (ESPE GmbH, Seefeld, Germany), glass ionomer cements, composite resins, intermediate restorative material (Caulk/Dentsply, Milford, DE), SuperEBA (Bosworth, Skokie, IL), and mineral trioxide aggregate (MTA; ProRoot MTA; Dentsply, Tulsa, OK).[20] Although none of these satisfy all the requirements of an ideal repair material, MTA has been the material of choice for root-end filling (**Fig. 4**E, F).

MTA was developed at Loma Linda University in the 1990s as a root-end filling material for endodontic surgery and is now indicated in many clinical settings. MTA demonstrates superior biocompatibility compared with other materials[21] and

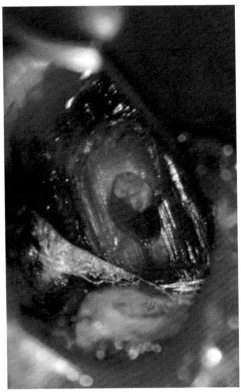

**Fig. 6.** Root-end preparation on a tooth #8. Ultrasonic root-end preparation resulted in a class I cavity coaxial to the root, with no debris or tissue remnants and no filling material left on the axial walls (magnification ×16).

promotes tissue regeneration when placed in contact with the periradicular tissues.[22]

Recently, a number of new bioactive materials based on tricalcium silicate cement have been introduced as potential root-end filling materials due to their ability to release calcium hydroxide in solution.[23] Such materials include Biodentine (Septodont, Saint-Maur-des-foss-es, France), Bioaggregate (Innovative Bioceramix Inc, Vancouver, Canada) and EndoSequence Root Repair Material (RRM) and Root Repair Putty (RRP) (Brasseler USA, Savannah GA) (see **Fig. 5**). According to manufacturers, both ERRM and ERRP are produced as premixed, homogeneous and consistent materials. Their physical properties include exceptional dimensional stability, high mechanical bond strength, high pH, and radiopaque and hydrophilic setting properties.[24] In vitro studies conclude that ERRM and ERRP have statistically similar levels of cytotoxicity to MTA, thus rendering them biocompatible materials for safe use.[24,25] Additional in vitro studies showed that bioceramic RRMs possess antibacterial properties[26] and sealing ability,[27] similar to those of MTA.

In a recent animal model study, RRM achieved a better tissue healing response adjacent to the resected root-end surface histologically compared with MTA. The superior healing tendency associated with RRM could be detected by CBCT and micro CT but not periapical radiography.[28]

The main differences between the traditional surgical technique and modern microsurgery are summarized in **Table 1**.

| Table 1 | | |
|---|---|---|
| Main differences between the traditional surgical technique and modern microsurgery | | |
| | Traditional Surgery | Microsurgery |
| Osteotomy size | 8–10 mm | 3–4 mm |
| Bevel angle degree | 45–65 | 0–10 |
| Inspection of resected surface | None | Always |
| Isthmus identification and treatment | Impossible | Always |
| Root-end preparation | Seldom inside canal | Always within canal |
| Root-end preparation instrument | Bur | Ultrasonic tips |
| Root-end filling material | Amalgam | Mineral trioxide triacetate |
| Sutures | 4 × 0 silk | 5 × 0, 6 × 0 monofilament |
| Suture removal | 7 d postoperative | 2–3 d postoperative |
| Healing success, 1-y follow-up | 40%–90% | 85%–97% |

*Modified from* Kim S, Kratchman S. Modern endodontic surgery concepts and practice: a review. J Endod 2006;32(7):602; with permission.

## MICROSURGICAL TECHNIQUE: PROGNOSIS AND TREATMENT OUTCOMES

Until a few years ago, endodontic surgery was faced with skepticism due to the insufficient knowledge of the apical anatomy as well as the reported limited success rate that the older surgical technique offered.

Modern microsurgical periradicular surgery uses certain technical advances, mainly the dental operating microscope, ultrasonics, modern microsurgical instruments, and biocompatible root-end filling materials and has obtained highly successful treatment outcomes.[29] These higher success rates were attributed to a superior inspection of the surgical site and to precise preparation of root-ends with microinstruments using high magnification and enhanced illumination.[30–32] The clinical success of microsurgically approached cases is reported to be as high as 96.8% and 91.5% at the short-term follow-up after 1 year and the long-term follow-up after 5 to 7 years, respectively.[6,33] Recent prospective studies with long-term follow-up have presented similar results.

To obtain a successful outcome in terms of healing of the existing periapical pathology, along with a good long-term prognosis in microsurgery, the strict case selection is of paramount importance. Kim and Kratchman[29] suggested a surgical classification A to F for proper case selection. Classes A to C were primarily endodontic lesions; classes D to F were cases with associated periodontal involvement. In a comparison of surgical outcome of these classes, Kim and colleagues[34] found a successful outcome of 95.2% for cases classified as A to C, compared with a success rate of 77.5% for classes D to F. Regenerative methods such as calcium sulfate and collagen membranes were used in the cases with a periodontal component in the pathology. Further investigation should be conducted in treatment of teeth with perio-endo communication via microsurgical and regenerative techniques. The current evidence though shows that microsurgery with regenerative techniques when indicated should be presented to the patient as a treatment option and a predictable and viable solution especially when the tooth is scheduled for an unnecessary extraction and implant placement.

## SUMMARY

With a high percentage of successful treatment outcomes of conventional endodontics together with high success of surgical endodontics, almost all teeth with endodontic lesions can be successfully treated. The challenge for the future will be the successful and predictable management of perio-endo lesions.

Further well-controlled experiments, clinical as well as biological, need to be conducted on many new techniques and materials to meet the present and future challenges. On the basis of published research, MTA is the material of choice for use in microsurgery, but new bioactive materials, such as bioceramic, seem to be equally reliable and probably more user friendly in clinical practice.

## REFERENCES

1. Kramper BJ, Kaminski EJ, Osetek EM, et al. A comparative study of the wound healing of three types of flap design used in periapical surgery. J Endod 1984; 10(1):17–25.
2. Velvart P. Papilla base incision: a new approach to recession-free healing of the interdental papilla after endodontic surgery. Int Endod J 2002;35(5):453–60.
3. Velvart P, Ebner-Zimmermann U, Ebner JP. Comparison of long-term papilla healing following sulcular full thickness flap and papilla base flap in endodontic surgery. Int Endod J 2004;37(10):687–93.
4. Rubinstein R. Magnification and illumination in apical surgery. Endod Top 2005; 11(1):56–77.
5. Kim S, Pecora G, Rubinstein R, editors. Color atlas of microsurgery in endodontics. Philadelphia: W.B. Saunders; 2001.
6. Rubinstein RA, Kim S. Short-term observation of the results of endodontic surgery with the use of a surgical operation microscope and Super-EBA as root-end filling material. J Endod 1999;25(1):43–8.
7. Carr GB. Microscope in endodontics. J Calif Dent Assoc 1992;20:55–61.
8. Cohen S, Burns R, editors. Pathways of the pulp. 6th edition. St Louis (MO): Mosby; 1994.
9. Rud J, Andreasen JO. A study of failures after endodontic surgery by radiographic, histologic and stereomicroscopic methods. Int J Oral Surg 1972;1(6): 311–28.
10. Gutmann JL, Harrison JW. Posterior endodontic surgery: anatomical considerations and clinical techniques. Int Endod J 1985;18(1):8–34.
11. Gutmann JL, Pitt Ford TR. Management of the resected root end: a clinical review. Int Endod J 1993;26(5):273–83.
12. Guttmann JL, Harrison JW, editors. Surgical endodontics. Boston: Blackwell Scientific Publications; 1991.
13. Cohen S, Burns R, editors. Pathways of the pulp. 8th edition. St Louis (MO): Mosby; 2002. p. 683–721.
14. Lubow RM, Wayman BE, Cooley RL. Endodontic flap design: analysis and recommendations for current usage. Oral Surg Oral Med Oral Pathol 1984;58(2): 207–12.
15. Weller RN, Niemczyk SP, Kim S. Incidence and position of the canal isthmus: part 1. Mesiobuccal root of the maxillary first molar. J Endod 1995;21(7):380–3.
16. Hsu YY, Kim S. The resected root surface. The issue of canal isthmuses. Dent Clin North Am 1997;41(3):529–40.
17. Nair PN, Henry S, Cano V, et al. Microbial status of apical root canal system of human mandibular first molars with primary apical periodontitis after "one-visit" endodontic treatment. Oral Surg Oral Med Oral Pathol Oral Radiol Endod 2005; 99(2):231–52.

18. Kim S. Principles of endodontic microsurgery. Dent Clin North Am 1997;41(3): 481–97.
19. Carr GB. Ultrasonic root end preparation. Dent Clin North Am 1997;41(3):541–4.
20. Torabinejad M, Pitt Ford TR. Root end filling materials: a review. Endod Dent Traumatol 1996;12(4):161–78.
21. Bodrumlu E. Biocompatibility of retrograde root filling materials: a review. Aust Endod J 2008;34(1):30–5.
22. Torabinejad M, Chivian N. Clinical applications of mineral trioxide aggregate. J Endod 1999;25(3):197–205.
23. Grech L, Mallia B, Camilleri J. Characterization of set intermediate restorative material, Biodentine, Bioaggregate and a prototype calcium silicate cement for use as root-end filling materials. Int Endod J 2013;46(7):632–41.
24. Damas BA, Wheater MA, Bringas JS, et al. Cytotoxicity comparison of mineral trioxide aggregates and Endosequence bioceramic root repair materials. J Endod 2011;37(3):372–5.
25. Hirschman WR, Wheater MA, Bringas JS, et al. Cytotoxicity comparison of three current direct pulp-capping agents with a new bioceramic root repair putty. J Endod 2012;38(3):385–8.
26. Lovato KF, Sedgley CM. Antibacterial activity of endosequence root repair material and proroot MTA against clinical isolates of Enterococcus faecalis. J Endod 2011;37(11):1542–6.
27. Nair U, Ghattas S, Saber M, et al. A comparative evaluation of the sealing ability of 2 root-end filling materials: an in vitro leakage study using Enterococcus faecalis. Oral Surg Oral Med Oral Pathol 2011;112(2):e74–7.
28. Chen I, Karabucak B, Wang C, et al. Healing after root-end microsurgery by using mineral trioxide aggregate and a new calcium silicate–based bioceramic material as root-end filling materials in dogs. J Endod 2015;41(3):389–99.
29. Kim S, Kratchman S. Modern endodontic surgery concepts and practice: a review. J Endod 2006;32(7):601–23.
30. Zuolo ML, Ferreira MO, Gutmann JL. Prognosis in periradicular surgery: a clinical prospective study. Int Endod J 2000;33(2):91–8.
31. Maddalone M, Gagliani M. Periapical endodontic surgery: a 3-year follow-up study. Int Endod J 2003;36(3):193–8.
32. Chong BS, Pitt Ford TR, Hudson MB. A prospective clinical study of mineral trioxide aggregate and IRM when used as root-end filling materials in endodontic surgery. Int Endod J 2003;35(8):520–6.
33. Rubinstein RA, Kim S. Long-term follow-up of cases considered healed one year after apical microsurgery. J Endod 2002;28(5):378–83.
34. Kim E, Song JS, Jung IY, et al. Prospective clinical study evaluating endodontic microsurgery outcomes for cases with lesions of endodontic origin compared with cases with lesions of combined periodontal-endodontic origin. J Endod 2008;34(5):546–51.

# Clinical and Molecular Perspectives of Reparative Dentin Formation

## Lessons Learned from Pulp-Capping Materials and the Emerging Roles of Calcium

Minju Song, DDS, PhD[a,b], Bo Yu, DDS, PhD[b], Sol Kim, PhD[a,b],
Marc Hayashi, DMD[b], Colby Smith, DDS[b], Suhjin Sohn, DDS, PhD[a],
Euiseong Kim, DDS, PhD[c], James Lim, DDS[b],
Richard G. Stevenson, DDS[b], Reuben H. Kim, DDS, PhD[a,b,*]

## KEYWORDS

- Reparative dentin • Calcium hydroxide • Hydraulic calcium-silicate cements
- Calcium • Odontoinductive • Odontoconductive • ORAI1

## KEY POINTS

- Direct pulp capping is often performed on the exposed pulp after deep caries removal to induce reparative dentin, a physical barrier that functions as a "biological seal" to protect the underlying pulp tissues and maintain pup vitality.
- Although calcium hydroxide (CH) has been used as the "gold standard" pulp-capping material for many decades, recently introduced hydraulic calcium-silicate cements (HCSCs), such as mineral trioxide aggregate (MTA), have increasingly gained popularity due to their superior material properties that are biocompatible, odontoconductive, and to a certain degree, odontoinductive.
- These pulp-capping materials confer capacity to induce reparative dentin by providing an alkaline environment and antibacterial activity; however, increasing lines of evidence support a notion that the release of calcium ions ($Ca^{2+}$) actively induces in reparative dentin formation by eliciting intracellular $Ca^{2+}$ signaling pathways.

*Continued*

---

Disclosure Statement: The authors declare that there is no conflict of interest related to this paper.
[a] The Shapiro Family Laboratory of Viral Oncology and Aging Research, UCLA School of Dentistry, 10833 Le Conte Avenue, Los Angeles, CA 90095, USA; [b] Section of Restorative Dentistry, UCLA School of Dentistry, 10833 Le Conte Avenue, Los Angeles, CA 90095, USA; [c] Microscope Center, Department of Conservative Dentistry, Oral Science Research Center, Yonsei University College of Dentistry, 50 Yonsei-Ro, 03772, Seoul, Korea
* Corresponding author. Center for the Health Sciences, UCLA School of Dentistry, Room 43-009, 10833 Le Conte Avenue, Los Angeles, CA 90095.
E-mail address: rkim@dentistry.ucla.edu

*Continued*

- Among the intracellular $Ca^{2+}$ regulators, ORAI1 protein was recently shown to have an indispensable role in odontogenic differentiation and mineralization in dental pulp stem cells by regulating $Ca^{2+}$ influx.
- Successful clinical outcomes of direct pulp capping depend on the operator technique, the material properties, and the host pulpal responses. Therefore, it is important to develop strategies that maximize the efficacy of each component for regenerating reparative dentin in a predictable and reproducible manner.

## INTRODUCTION

Dental caries is the most prevalent infectious oral disease experienced by more than 90% of adults in the United States.[1,2] A quarter of US populations do not have dental insurance,[3] and more than 60% of underserved areas are still in need of dentists.[4] Considering these potentially unidentified individuals, it is expected that almost all individuals may have experienced dental caries at least once in their lifetime.

Due to its high prevalence, removing dental caries is one of the most common procedures performed in routine dental practices. During caries removal, deep caries penetrating through the enamel and dentin frequently leads to either indirect or direct pulp-capping procedures to induce tertiary (reactionary or reparative, respectively) dentin formation.[5] Several pulp-capping materials, including calcium hydroxide (Ca [OH]$_2$ or CH) and hydraulic calcium-silicate cements (HCSCs), such as mineral trioxide aggregate (MTA), are used for this purpose. For indirect pulp capping, these materials are placed on the "unexposed" pulp to enhance reactionary dentin formation from the existing odontoblasts at the dentino-pulpal complex. In contrast, direct pulp capping refers to placing the pulp-capping materials on the "exposed" pulp, where odontoblast layers are breached, to enhance reparative dentin formation mediated by odontoblast-like cells differentiated from dental pulp stem cells (DPSCs) at the materio-pulpal complex (MPC).

Unlike indirect pulp capping, which usually has predictable clinical outcomes, direct pulp capping has outcomes that are often variable depending on the operator technique, the material properties, and the host pulpal responses. In direct pulp capping, the ultimate goal is to preserve the underlying pulp and maintain pulp vitality by regenerating reparative dentin at the MPC, which functions as a "biological seal" to protect the underlying pulp tissues, to increase the life expectancy of the tooth, and to improve the overall oral health. A successful pulp-capping procedure can avoid more invasive and expensive dental treatment, such as root canal therapy. Therefore, it is important to optimize direct pulp-capping techniques, improve biocompatibility of the materials, and enhance biological responses of the pulp tissues to maximize regeneration of reparative dentin.

Here, we discuss the current status of different types of direct pulp-capping materials with specific focuses on CH and HCSCs due to their extensive clinical utilization and substantial amounts of available studies. We then attempt to delineate molecular mechanisms by which reparative dentin forms based on the common properties of these pulp-capping materials, as well as known bone-grafting materials. Finally, we suggest possible roles of calcium ions ($Ca^{2+}$) in the formation of mineralized tissues, including reparative dentin and bone.

## CLINICAL PERSPECTIVES: PULP-CAPPING MATERIALS IN PULPAL THERAPY
### *Calcium Hydroxide*

CH was first introduced to the dental profession in 1920s, and has long been recognized as the gold standard pulp-capping material.[6–8] Early clinical studies including more than 2300 cases of direct pulp capping showed 80% to 90% success rate.[6] Recent review of literature revealed that the overall success rates, as mostly determined by an asymptomatic tooth without radiographic lesions, fall between 68.5% and 80.1% within a 2-year follow-up period but drops to 58.7% to 76.3% after 10 years.[9–12] As such, the use of CH as a direct pulp-capping material is frequently performed (**Fig. 1**).

One of the most clinically relevant functions of CH is the facilitation of reparative dentin formation. Histologic studies of pulp-capped teeth revealed a thin layer of coagulation necrosis in the pulp due to the irrigation from high pH.[8,13] Mild inflammation, cellular debris, and calcium-protein granules were observed below the superficial necrotic layer onto which the eventual dentin bridge formed. Although detailed mechanisms remain elusive, the superficial necrosis was believed to be vital for initiation of dentin-bridge formation.[7,13–15] It was also suggested that CH facilitates reparative

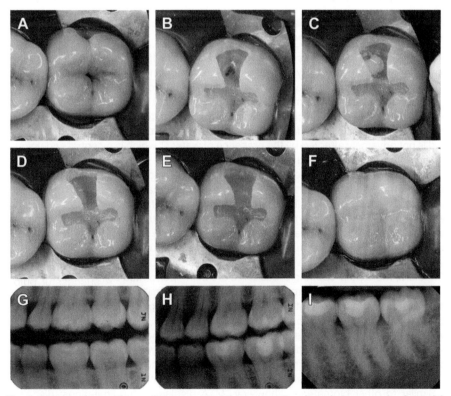

**Fig. 1.** Direct pulp capping on #18 using CH. (*A*) Preoperative clinical photograph of #18. (*B*) bucco-occlusal preparation with exposed mesio-buccal pulp horn. (*C*) Dycal placement on the exposed pulp. (*D*) Fuji Lining LC placement as a liner directly on Dycal. (*E*) Fuji II LC placed as a base on #18 on top of Dycal. (*F*) Composite restoration on #18. (*G*) Preoperative radiograph of #18. (*H*) Postoperative radiograph of #18. (*I*) Periapical radiograph of #18 at follow-up after 2.5 years.

dentin formation through the creation of an alkaline environment and an increased availability of calcium ions.[7,13,16,17]

However, there are several disadvantages. CH dressings dissolve clinically within 1 to 2 years.[18,19] The susceptibility to dissolution by acid and tissue fluid presented a problem during subsequent acid-etch resin restoration.[20] CH lacks inherent adhesion to dentin, but in newer formulations, may bind to dentin via urethane dimethacrylate, which also partially adds resistance to acid dissolution.[21] The most prominent issue with CH is that 89% of dentin bridges formed contained tunnel defects.[19,22] Considering that the dissolution of the dressing leaves a void beneath the restoration, these "tunnel defects" present a high risk for microleakage, leading to bacterial reinfection, persisting pulpal inflammation, and necrosis. These disadvantages may potentially be linked to notable variation in outcomes and a decrease in clinical success rate over follow-up time.[9,10] Consistent with such notions, numerous studies reported that the success rate of pulp capping with CH varies significantly, ranging from 13% to 95%.[23–25]

In summary, CH remains favored by practitioners for pulpal therapy due to its excellent antimicrobial activity and capacity to form reparative dentin. However, tunnel defects and progressive dissolution compromise the integrity of reparative dentin, and these shortfalls call into questions the use of CH as a long-term pulp therapeutic agent.

### Hydraulic Calcium-Silicate Cements

MTA, a prototype HCSC, was first introduced in the early 1990s by Torabinejad and his coworkers.[26,27] It was initially recommended as a root-end filling material but subsequently used in various clinical applications, such as pulp capping, pulpotomy, apexogenesis, apical barrier formation, and repair of root perforations.[28] The main composition of MTA is tricalcium silicate, dicalcium silicate, tricalcium aluminate, bismuth oxide, and calcium sulfate dehydrate. MTA is hygroscopic; its setting requires and is not adversely affected by the presence of water,[29] which is a central and unique advantage that contrasts with existing dental materials.

Increasing lines of evidence support a notion that MTA confers superior clinical outcomes. Although some reports showed insignificant clinical outcomes with MTA when compared with CH,[30] other clinical studies showed more favorable success rates with MTA than CH.[12,31–33] In some of these studies, the success rates of direct pulp capping using MTA have been reported to exceed more than 90%.[34–36] In addition, success rates seem to be maintained over long follow-up periods with MTA,[32,36,37] which was different from CHs that show time-dependent decline in success rates.[38,39] Therefore, more pulp-capping procedures are being performed using HCSCs (**Fig. 2**).

The superior clinical outcomes of MTA are attributed to its physical properties: flexural strength, compressive strength, and push-out strength, as well as antimicrobial effect, radiopacity, dimensional stability, and tolerance to moisture.[40] In addition, MTA has shown to have better sealing properties,[29,41] biocompatibility,[42,43] and osteogenic/odontogenic differentiation capacity.[44,45] As the type of pulp-capping material was shown to be the single most important factor influencing the pulpal survival rate among others,[33] these properties contribute to its favorable clinical outcomes.

Similar to other biomaterials, however, MTA displays some limitations: discoloration, long setting time, difficulty in manipulation, and high cost.[28] A long setting time (eg, 2 hours 45 minutes) is one of the major drawbacks of MTA, which may delay the completion of the treatment in a single appointment in the clinic. Indeed, the prototype MTA requires temporization of the tooth to achieve the proper hardness before final restoration, which creates another potential problem of microleakage or

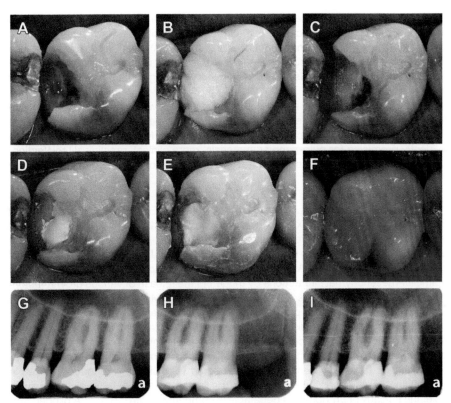

**Fig. 2.** Direct pulp capping on #14 using HCSCs. (*A*) Disto-occlusal preparation with exposed pulp. (*B*) Cotton pellet soaked with 3.5% NaOCl. (*C*) Hemostasis achieved at the pulp-exposed area. (*D*) Placement of bioceramics on the exposed pulp. (*E*) Fuji Plus placement as base directly on the HCSCs. (*F*) Composite restoration on #14. (*G*) Preoperative radiograph of #14. (*H*) Postoperative radiograph of #14. (*I*) Periapical radiograph of #14 at the follow-up after 1.5 years.

reinfection while the temporary is in place.[46] Discoloration is another major drawback, especially when it is used on the anterior teeth, requiring additional treatment such as bleaching.[47] A tooth-colored white MTA was developed to overcome this limitation; however, unexpected tooth discoloration has also been reported by this white MTA.[48,49] Furthermore, handling of MTA is another challenge for clinicians, which potentially discourages its routine use in clinical applications.

In 2013, the original patent for the prototype MTA was expired, and since then, a number of different HCSCs were introduced. Similar to MTA, these materials share common physicochemical and biocompatible properties but are claimed to have improved characteristics.[50] For example, Biodentine (Septodont, Saint-Maur-des-Fosses, France) and Endocem (Maruchi, Wonju, Korea) are fast-setting HCSCs with the setting time of 12.0 minutes and 4.5 minutes, respectively. Biodentine has a shortened setting time with the addition of a setting accelerator ($CaCl_2$) and the removal of the liquid component,[51] whereas Endocem has small particle sizes that increase surface contact with water, resulting in fast setting and ease of manipulation.[52] Another improvement is the replacement of the opacifier with bismuth oxide to zirconium oxide.[53,54] Because bismuth oxide causes MTA discoloration after light irradiation in an oxygen-free environment,[55] the zirconium oxide–containing HCSCs, such as Endocem, RetroMTA

(BioMTA, Seoul, Korea), Biodentine, and Endosequence (Brasseler USA, Savannah, GA) are suggested as better choices for esthetic reasons. Additional improvement includes better handling properties; Endosequence (Brasseler USA) is a premixed, ready-to-use syringeable paste that is condensable, which make them user friendly with an ease of handling and application. It also has a demonstrated strength and biologic effect similar to MTA.[56]

Despite the rapid increase in newly developed HCSCs with multiple modifications in their compositions, there are insufficient studies to experimentally support whether they are superior or even comparable alternatives to MTA. Although HCSCs are evidently promising for pulp-capping materials, more clinical, preclinical, and molecular studies are needed to define the clinical efficacy for regenerating the pulp for reparative dentin formation.

### Emdogain

Emdogain is an enamel matrix derivative (EMD) product extracted from the Hertwig root sheath during porcine tooth development. Originally developed to promote regeneration of periodontium,[57] Emdogain has been proposed in several recent studies as a potential pulp-capping material.[58,59] Amelogenins, the major components of EMD, can mimic epithelial-mesenchymal interactions by triggering the release of various growth factors and cytokines, such as bone morphogenetic protein (BMP) and transforming growth factor (TGF)-$\beta$, which in turn promote differentiation of mesenchymal stem cells in the pulp into odontoblast-like cells.[60,61] In addition, EMD may also enhance dentin mineralization, as odontoblast-like cells reportedly upregulate mineralization-inducing genes on treatment with Emdogain.[62] In the context of pulp capping, EMD may facilitate formation of thicker reparative dentin barrier compared with CH, as was indeed proven in several animal studies.[63,64] However, with the limited number of human studies available, the efficacy of Emdogain is debatable in comparison with CH.[65–67] A blinded randomized clinical study on experimentally exposed human pulp showed ineffective hard tissue barrier formation by Emdogain, although postoperative symptoms were less frequent compared with CH.[66] More pulpal inflammation was also associated with Emdogain treatment. Two other studies on primary teeth,[67] and partial pulpotomy in permanent teeth,[65] failed to establish superiority of reparative dentin formation by Emdogain. Of note, these studies consisted of a limited sample size (<45 subjects) and short follow-up period (3–12 months). Hence, the clinical efficacy and safety of Emdogain as a pulp-capping material is inconclusive at best and requires further investigation.

### Growth Factors and Matrix-Derived Proteins

Since the turn of the century, several bioactive materials for pulp-capping alternatives have been proposed and have been reviewed elsewhere.[68] Growth factors (BMPs, insulin-like growth factor-1, epidermal growth factor, fibroblast growth factor, TGF, platelet-derived growth factor) and matrix-derived proteins (bone sialoprotein) may stimulate reparative dentin formation that is comparable or even superior to CH, but appropriate delivery carrier and dosage need to be considered for controlled reparative dentin regeneration. The limited half-life also necessitates the need for multiple applications, which may incur high cost. As such, studies for efficacies of these bioactive molecules in pulp capping remain to be determined in the in vitro and animal study stages.

## MOLECULAR PERSPECTIVES: COMMON PROPERTIES OF PULP-CAPPING MATERIALS

Pulpal wound healing including reparative dentin formation is a multifactorial, complex process that is orchestrated by discrete but overlapping steps of migration, proliferation, and mineralization of pulp cells.[69] Unlike reactionary dentin, which is formed by existing odontoblasts, reparative dentin is formed by odontoblast-like cells presumably differentiated from DPSCs when the pulp becomes exposed and the existing odontoblastic layers are breached. At the cellular level, these DPSCs are expected to migrate to and proliferate on the MPC, ultimately undergoing odontogenic differentiation to form reparative dentin.

Although both CH and HCSCs are thought to be odontoconductive by functioning as scaffolds for proper execution of these processes by DPSCs, clinical and molecular studies suggest evidently that they are also odontoinductive, such that these materials can stimulate DPSCs to undergo odontogenic differentiation and mineralization. Therefore, identifying the factors released from pulp-capping agents that regulate DPSCs to form reparative dentin and defining the fundamental molecular mechanisms by which DPSCs respond to these pulp-capping agents are critically important for regenerating reparative dentin and creating a "biological seal."

As was discussed previously, there exist a number of pulp-capping materials that are clinically proven to induce reparative dentin formation in humans. Based on this historical evidence, some of the properties are suggested to play key roles in regenerating reparative dentin. These properties include the following:

1. High pH
2. Antibacterial activity
3. Calcium ion release

### High pH

Alkaline environment (high pH) is known to promote osteogenic differentiation and bone formation.[70,71] Conversely, acidic environment is demonstrated to inhibit bone formation.[72] Alkaline phosphatase, an important enzyme in initiating calcification, allows for the increase in local concentration of inorganic phosphate at an alkaline pH.[73] Because CH is a water-soluble compound that dissolves on contact with tissue fluid and releases hydroxyl anions ($OH^-$) to increase pH to 12 to 13, it was suggested that such alkaline pH attributes to reparative dentin formation by CH.[74–76] Similarly, HCSCs also were demonstrated to create a high-pH environment, as the end product of the chemical reaction is CH.[77–79]

Although an alkaline environment is essential for creating an osteoinductive environment, mineralization is highly sensitive to pH change; alkaline phosphatase activity peaks at pH 7.37 and significantly diminished above this physiologic level.[72] Furthermore, pH above 8.0 was shown to inhibit mineralization process both in vitro and in vivo.[80,81] Because measuring the precise pH at or around the interfaces between pulp-capping materials and pulp tissue is technically challenging, further investigation is needed to clarify the actual effects of high pH on reparative dentin formation in vivo.

### Antimicrobial Activity

One of the clinical advantages of CH as a pulp medicament largely derives from its antimicrobial activity due to $OH^-$ release (pH up to 12.5). The highly reactive hydroxyl radicals along with the raised pH can cause damage to the cytoplasmic membrane and DNA of bacterial microorganisms.[82,83] In addition, the high pH may also provide anti-inflammatory effects, via denaturation of proinflammatory cytokines[84] and stimulation of regulatory interleukin-10.[85] Sustained attenuation of bacterial irritation and inflammatory response in turn may provide a conductive environment for reparative dentin formation. However, such effects are indirect; the removal of bacterial organisms does not actively contribute to reparative dentin formation. Therefore, it remains to be elucidated whether antimicrobial activity of the dental pulp-capping materials is a molecular determinant in reparative dentin formation.

### Calcium Ions

Although $Ca^{2+}$ is one of the major constituents released by both CH and HCSCs,[77,86] the role of $Ca^{2+}$ in reparative dentin formation is largely underexplored. An earlier study demonstrated that, when CH with radiolabeled $Ca^{2+}$ was used as a direct pulp-capping material on pulp-exposed teeth in dogs, radiocalcium was not found in the reparative dentin area, suggesting that $Ca^{2+}$ necessary for formation of reparative dentin matrix itself is not derived from CH but from the pulp.[87] However, emerging evidence supports a notion that $Ca^{2+}$ plays indispensable roles not only in formation of mineralized matrixes but also in transduction of the intracellular signaling pathway that are involved in maintaining and regulating normal biological processes.[88,89] Indeed, recent studies suggested that $Ca^{2+}$ released from biomaterials is one of the key factors mediating mineralization process[7,86] and that $Ca^{2+}$ released from pulp-capping materials may be an active component in reparative dentin formation.

Unlike its role in dentin formation, $Ca^{2+}$ in bone formation is well documented. High amounts of extracellular $Ca^{2+}$ induced expression of alkaline phosphatase (ALP), osteocalcin (OC), and osteopontin (OP) in pre-osteoblast cells.[90,91] Furthermore, extracellular $Ca^{2+}$ also induced osteoblast differentiation and mineralization both in vitro and in vivo,[92–94] indicating that $Ca^{2+}$ alone has a de novo characteristic to induce osteogenic differentiation.

To enhance bone formation in vivo, biomaterials such as hydroxyapatite (HA), tricalcium phosphates (TCP), or biphasic calcium phosphates (BCP), a mixture of HA and TCP, are frequently used as scaffolds for bone grafting.[95] Although these materials are known to be osteoconductive in nature by serving as scaffold for bone growth, they are also suggested to be osteoinductive; these materials by themselves actively stimulate differentiation of pre-osteoblastic cells to osteoblasts and formation of new bone.[96,97] Interestingly, all of these materials are highly enriched with $Ca^{2+}$,[98] and their capacity to induce bone formation seems to differ depending on the amount of $Ca^{2+}$. Indeed, Ca/P ratio of TCP is 1.67 when that of HA is 1.5, and TCP is capable of releasing more $Ca^{2+}$ than HA.[99] Furthermore, Barradas and colleagues[100] demonstrated that TCP induces more bone formation than HA both in vitro and in vivo, and such difference is primarily attributed to high solubility of TCP to release $Ca^{2+}$.

Similar to osteoblasts, extracellular $Ca^{2+}$ also induces odontogenic differentiation of dental mesenchymal cells. $Ca^{2+}$ treatment alone induced osteogenic gene expression, such as osteopontin and BMP2 in dental pulp cells.[101,102] Mizuno and Banzai[103] also showed that $Ca^{2+}$ released from CH stimulated fibronectin gene expression in dental pulp cells, a mechanism that may induce differentiation of these cells to become mineralized-tissue–forming cells. Elevated $Ca^{2+}$ is also known to stimulate differentiation and mineralization of other dental mesenchymal cells, such as cementoblasts, by increasing FGF-2 expression.[104]

At the molecular level, extracellular $Ca^{2+}$ level is detected by the calcium-sensing receptor (CaSR), a 7-transmembrane homodimer receptor that belongs to the C family of the G-protein–coupled receptor superfamily. An activated CaSR elicits intracellular signaling pathways that ultimately lead to migration, proliferation, and differentiation of cells.[105] Recently, it was shown that CaSR mediates osteogenic differentiation and mineralization of bone marrow mesenchymal stromal cells.[106] However, the presence of CaSR in bone-forming cells is controversial,[107] and osteoblasts derived from

CaSR-null mice remained to possess osteogenic differentiation potential.[108,109] Further, another study demonstrated that inhibition of CaSR further induced, rather than suppressed, $Ca^{2+}$-mediated osteogenic differentiation,[110] suggesting that CaSR is dispensable in osteogenic differentiation and mineralization.

$Ca^{2+}$ itself is an important intracellular signaling molecule, and there exist different types of $Ca^{2+}$ channels that regulate intracellular $Ca^{2+}$ level.[111] Among them, L-type voltage-gated calcium channel was shown to be associated with $Ca^{2+}$-mediated osteogenic differentiation and mineralization.[112–115] Similarly, recent studies showed that L-type calcium channel plays a key role in differentiation of DPSCs and periodontal ligament cells.[110,116] However, L-type voltage-gated calcium channel is a large transmembrane multiprotein complex that mediates $Ca^{2+}$ influx in response to membrane depolarization via voltage differences.[111] As such, it remains to be elucidated as to how membrane depolarization links to differentiation and mineralization of osteoblasts and odontoblasts.

Recent studies identified another class of calcium channel, ORAI1 that regulates intracellular $Ca^{2+}$ level and $Ca^{2+}$-mediated signaling pathway in most nonexcitable cells.[117] ORAI1 is an essential subunit of $Ca^{2+}$ release–activated $Ca^{2+}$ (CRAC) channel that mediates $Ca^{2+}$ influx via the store-operated $Ca^{2+}$ entry (SOCE) mechanism. Although ORAI1 is extensively studied and characterized in immune cells,[118] recent studies showed that it plays a critical role in mediating bone formation. In particular, Orai1-null mice exhibited osteoporotic phenotypes, and disruption of ORAI1 function in osteoblasts suppressed osteogenic differentiation and mineralization.[119–121] Similarly, Sohn and colleagues[122] recently demonstrated that ORAI1 also plays an indispensable role in odontogenic differentiation and mineralization. When ORAI1 was knocked down in DPSCs, these cells exhibited not only incompetent $Ca^{2+}$ influx (**Fig. 3**) but also inability to undergo odontogenic differentiation and mineralization as demonstrated by alkaline phosphatase staining and activity as well as alizarin red staining (see **Fig. 3**). More importantly, transplantation of DPSCs harboring Orai1/E106Q, a dominant negative form of ORAI1 caused no formation of mineralized nodules in vivo, indicating that ORAI1 is required for odontogenic differentiation and mineralization both in vitro and in vivo. Further studies on the role of ORAI1 in reparative dentin formation warrant closer examination.

## SUMMARY

Although a substantial numbers of clinical and molecular studies support the use of CH and HCSCs for direct pulp capping, achieving clinically successful outcomes in a reproducible and reliable manner still requires more investigations. Such shortfalls may be due, in part, to the lack of thorough understanding in the fundamental mechanisms of pulpal wound healing and reparative dentin formation. Many pulp-capping animal models were previously used to better understand the mechanisms of reparative dentin formation[123–125]; however, pulp-capping studies in large animals are usually observational in nature. For this reason, transgenic or knockout mice that have an overexpressed or deleted gene of interest in an inducible and cell-type specific manner would help in expediting our understanding in reparative dentin formation at the molecular level.[126,127]

Due to the favorable clinical outcomes with the prototype MTA, its derivative products are widely available with modifications to their compositions. Nonetheless, their relative efficacy, or even their toxicity, is still far from complete understanding. Further comparative studies on validating and standardizing the effects of different HCSCs also warrant closer examination.

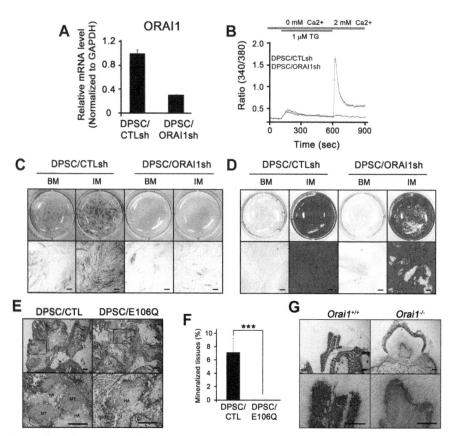

**Fig. 3.** The calcium channel, ORAI1, plays an indispensable role in odontogenic differentiation and mineralization. (*A*) Quantitative real-time polymerase chain reaction (qRT-PCR) of ORAI1 expression following knockdown experiment in DPSCs, showing efficient suppression of ORAI1 in DPSC/ORAI1sh cells but not in DPSC/CTLsh cells. (*B*) Measurement of intracellular $Ca^{2+}$ level in DPSCs, confirming inhibition of $Ca^{2+}$ influx when ORAI1 expression is suppressed in DPSCs. (*C*) Alkaline phosphatase (ALP) staining of DPSCs following treatment with basal medium (BM) and bone-forming induction medium (IM) for 5 days, demonstrating inhibition of ALP activity important for odontogenic differentiation. (*D*) Alizarin red staining of DPSCs following treatment with BM and bone-forming IM for 14 days, demonstrating inhibition of odontogenic mineralization. (*E*) Ectopic mineralized-tissue formation of DPSC/CTL cells but not DPSC/E106Q cells harboring dominant negative form of ORAI1, demonstrating indispensable role of ORAI1 in vivo. (*F*) Quantification of ectopic mineralized-tissue formation in vivo (***, p < 0.0005). (*G*) ALP staining of a tooth prepared from *Orai1*$^{+/+}$ and *Orai1*$^{-/-}$ mice. (*From* Sohn S, Park Y, Srikanth S, et al. The role of ORAI1 in the odontogenic differentiation of human dental pulp stem cells. J Dent Res 2015;94(11); 1564, 1566.)

CH and HCSCs are odontoconductive by functioning as scaffolds onto which DPSCs migrate, proliferate, and differentiate to form reparative dentin. Clinical and preclinical studies support a notion that they are also odontoinductive, as they also stimulate DPSCs to form reparative dentin (**Fig. 4**). It would be beneficial and effective to incorporate bioactive materials as one of their constituents to further potentiate odontoconductive and odontoinductive properties of the pulp-capping materials.

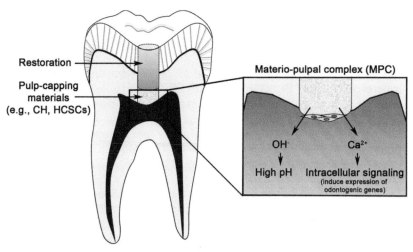

**Fig. 4.** Schematic diagram of molecular mechanisms that govern reparative dentin formation by CH or HCSCs at the MPC. CH and HCSCs release hydroxyl group ($OH^-$) and increase local pH at the MPC, creating an alkaline environment that induces antibacterial activity and potentially promotes odontogenic mineralization. CH and HCSCs also release calcium ions ($Ca^{2+}$), eliciting intracellular signaling pathways that ultimately promote odontogenic differentiation and mineralization.

Historically, CH has been used as a pulp-capping material, and its efficacy has proven to protect the exposed pulp based on clinical experiences for many decades. Recently introduced HCSCs have increasingly gained popularity due to improved physical and chemical properties to enhance reparative dentin formation. Nonetheless, many practitioners still prefer complete removal of the pulp once exposed rather than pulp-capping placement, primarily due to apprehension that they would be perceived as an "incompetent dentist" for the unsuccessful outcomes and multiple subsequent visits should the pulp capping fail. Because successful direct pulp capping is largely dependent on operator technique, material properties, and the host pulpal responses, it is important to recognize the importance of, and to optimally maximize the merits of each component so that reparative dentin can be regenerated in a predictable and reproducible manner. In this regard, more studies are needed at the clinical, preclinical, and molecular levels to improve each component.

## ACKNOWLEDGMENTS

This study was, in part, supported by grants from NIDCR/NIH R01DE023348 (RHK), UCLA Faculty Research grant (RHK), and Dean's Faculty Research Seed grant (RHK).

## REFERENCES

1. Dye B, Thornton-Evans G, Li X, et al. Dental caries and tooth loss in adults in the United States, 2011-2012. NCHS Data Brief 2015;(197):197.
2. Dye BA, Tan S, Smith V, et al. Trends in oral health status: United States, 1988-1994 and 1999-2004. Vital Health Stat 11 2007;(248):1–92.
3. Bloom B, Cohen RA. Dental insurance for persons under age 65 years with private health insurance: United States, 2008. NCHS Data Brief 2010;(40):1–8.

4. Statistics DHPSA. First Quarter of Fiscal Year 2016 Designated HPSA Quarterly Summary. Bureau of Health Workforce Health Resources and Services Administration (HRSA) U.S. Department of Health & Human Services, www.hhs.gov, 2015.

5. Goldberg M, Kulkarni AB, Young M, et al. Dentin: structure, composition and mineralization. Front Biosci (Elite Ed) 2011;3:711–35.

6. Baume LJ, Holz J. Long term clinical assessment of direct pulp capping. Int Dent J 1981;31(4):251–60.

7. Sangwan P, Sangwan A, Duhan J, et al. Tertiary dentinogenesis with calcium hydroxide: a review of proposed mechanisms. Int Endod J 2013;46(1):3–19.

8. Hilton TJ. Keys to clinical success with pulp capping: a review of the literature. Oper Dent 2009;34(5):615–25.

9. Willershausen B, Willershausen I, Ross A, et al. Retrospective study on direct pulp capping with calcium hydroxide. Quintessence Int 2011;42(2):165–71.

10. Dammaschke T, Leidinger J, Schafer E. Long-term evaluation of direct pulp capping–treatment outcomes over an average period of 6.1 years. Clin Oral Investig 2010;14(5):559–67.

11. Matsuo T, Nakanishi T, Shimizu H, et al. A clinical study of direct pulp capping applied to carious-exposed pulps. J Endod 1996;22(10):551–6.

12. Hilton TJ, Ferracane JL, Mancl L. Northwest practice-based research collaborative in evidence-based D. Comparison of CaOH with MTA for direct pulp capping: a PBRN randomized clinical trial. J Dent Res 2013;92(7 Suppl): 16S–22S.

13. Estrela C, Sydney GB, Bammann LL, et al. Mechanism of action of calcium and hydroxyl ions of calcium hydroxide on tissue and bacteria. Braz Dent J 1995; 6(2):85–90.

14. Estrela C, Pimenta FC, Ito IY, et al. Antimicrobial evaluation of calcium hydroxide in infected dentinal tubules. J Endod 1999;25(6):416–8.

15. Holland R, de Souza V, Nery MJ, et al. Reaction of rat connective tissue to implanted dentin tubes filled with mineral trioxide aggregate or calcium hydroxide. J Endod 1999;25(3):161–6.

16. Okabe T, Sakamoto M, Takeuchi H, et al. Effects of pH on mineralization ability of human dental pulp cells. J Endod 2006;32(3):198–201.

17. Foreman PC, Barnes IE. Review of calcium hydroxide. Int Endod J 1990;23(6): 283–97.

18. Stanley HR, Pameijer CH. Pulp capping with a new visible-light-curing calcium hydroxide composition (Prisma VLC Dycal). Oper Dent 1985;10(4):156–63.

19. Cox CF, Bergenholtz G, Heys DR, et al. Pulp capping of dental pulp mechanically exposed to oral microflora: a 1-2 year observation of wound healing in the monkey. J Oral Pathol 1985;14(2):156–68.

20. Olmez A, Oztas N, Basak F, et al. A histopathologic study of direct pulp-capping with adhesive resins. Oral Surg Oral Med Oral Pathol Oral Radiol Endod 1998; 86(1):98–103.

21. Pameijer CH, Stanley HR. The disastrous effects of the "total etch" technique in vital pulp capping in primates. Am J Dent 1998;11 Spec No:S45–54.

22. Cox CF, Subay RK, Ostro E, et al. Tunnel defects in dentin bridges: their formation following direct pulp capping. Oper Dent 1996;21(1):4–11.

23. Al-Hiyasat AS, Barrieshi-Nusair KM, Al-Omari MA. The radiographic outcomes of direct pulp-capping procedures performed by dental students: a retrospective study. J Am Dent Assoc 2006;137(12):1699–705.

24. Barthel CR, Rosenkranz B, Leuenberg A, et al. Pulp capping of carious exposures: treatment outcome after 5 and 10 years: a retrospective study. J Endod 2000;26(9):525–8.
25. Cvek M. A clinical report on partial pulpotomy and capping with calcium hydroxide in permanent incisors with complicated crown fracture. J Endod 1978;4(8): 232–7.
26. Ford TR, Torabinejad M, Abedi HR, et al. Using mineral trioxide aggregate as a pulp-capping material. J Am Dent Assoc 1996;127(10):1491–4.
27. Torabinejad M, Watson TF, Pitt Ford TR. Sealing ability of a mineral trioxide aggregate when used as a root end filling material. J Endod 1993;19(12):591–5.
28. Parirokh M, Torabinejad M. Mineral trioxide aggregate: a comprehensive literature review–Part III: clinical applications, drawbacks, and mechanism of action. J Endod 2010;36(3):400–13.
29. Torabinejad M, Higa RK, McKendry DJ, et al. Dye leakage of four root end filling materials: effects of blood contamination. J Endod 1994;20(4):159–63.
30. Iwamoto CE, Adachi E, Pameijer CH, et al. Clinical and histological evaluation of white ProRoot MTA in direct pulp capping. Am J Dent 2006;19(2):85–90.
31. Nair PN, Duncan HF, Pitt Ford TR, et al. Histological, ultrastructural and quantitative investigations on the response of healthy human pulps to experimental capping with Mineral Trioxide Aggregate: a randomized controlled trial. 2008. Int Endod J 2009;42(5):422–44.
32. Mente J, Geletneky B, Ohle M, et al. Mineral trioxide aggregate or calcium hydroxide direct pulp capping: an analysis of the clinical treatment outcome. J Endod 2010;36(5):806–13.
33. Cho SY, Seo DG, Lee SJ, et al. Prognostic factors for clinical outcomes according to time after direct pulp capping. J Endod 2013;39(3):327–31.
34. Marques MS, Wesselink PR, Shemesh H. Outcome of direct pulp capping with mineral trioxide aggregate: a prospective study. J Endod 2015;41(7):1026–31.
35. Farsi N, Alamoudi N, Balto K, et al. Clinical assessment of mineral trioxide aggregate (MTA) as direct pulp capping in young permanent teeth. J Clin Pediatr Dent 2006;31(2):72–6.
36. Bogen G, Kim JS, Bakland LK. Direct pulp capping with mineral trioxide aggregate: an observational study. J Am Dent Assoc 2008;139(3):305–15 [quiz: 305–15].
37. Jang Y, Song M, Yoo IS, et al. A randomized controlled study of the use of proroot mineral trioxide aggregate and endocem as direct pulp capping materials: 3-month versus 1-year outcomes. J Endod 2015;41(8):1201–6.
38. Horsted P, Sandergaard B, Thylstrup A, et al. A retrospective study of direct pulp capping with calcium hydroxide compounds. Endod Dent Traumatol 1985;1(1):29–34.
39. Haskell EW, Stanley HR, Chellemi J, et al. Direct pulp capping treatment: a long-term follow-up. J Am Dent Assoc 1978;97(4):607–12.
40. Parirokh M, Torabinejad M. Mineral trioxide aggregate: a comprehensive literature review–Part I: chemical, physical, and antibacterial properties. J Endod 2010;36(1):16–27.
41. Torabinejad M, Smith PW, Kettering JD, et al. Comparative investigation of marginal adaptation of mineral trioxide aggregate and other commonly used root-end filling materials. J Endod 1995;21(6):295–9.
42. Camilleri J, Montesin FE, Di Silvio L, et al. The chemical constitution and biocompatibility of accelerated Portland cement for endodontic use. Int Endod J 2005; 38(11):834–42.

43. Torabinejad M, Parirokh M. Mineral trioxide aggregate: a comprehensive litera-ture review–part II: leakage and biocompatibility investigations. J Endod 2010; 36(2):190–202.

44. Seo MS, Hwang KG, Lee J, et al. The effect of mineral trioxide aggregate on odontogenic differentiation in dental pulp stem cells. J Endod 2013;39(2):242–8.

45. Wang Y, Yan M, Fan Z, et al. Mineral trioxide aggregate enhances the odonto/osteogenic capacity of stem cells from inflammatory dental pulps via NF-kappaB pathway. Oral Dis 2014;20(7):650–8.

46. Song M, Kang M, Kim HC, et al. A randomized controlled study of the use of ProRoot mineral trioxide aggregate and Endocem as direct pulp capping mate-rials. J Endod 2015;41(1):11–5.

47. Jang JH, Kang M, Ahn S, et al. Tooth discoloration after the use of new pozzolan cement (endocem) and mineral trioxide aggregate and the effects of internal bleaching. J Endod 2013;39(12):1598–602.

48. Belobrov I, Parashos P. Treatment of tooth discoloration after the use of white mineral trioxide aggregate. J Endod 2011;37(7):1017–20.

49. Lenherr P, Allgayer N, Weiger R, et al. Tooth discoloration induced by endodon-tic materials: a laboratory study. Int Endod J 2012;45(10):942–9.

50. Dawood AE, Parashos P, Wong RHK, et al. Calcium silicate-based cements: composition, properties, and clinical applications. J Investig Clin Dent 2015;0: 1–15.

51. Nayak G, Hasan MF. Biodentine-a novel dentinal substitute for single visit apex-ification. Restor Dent Endod 2014;39(2):120–5.

52. Choi Y, Park SJ, Lee SH, et al. Biological effects and washout resistance of a newly developed fast-setting pozzolan cement. J Endod 2013;39(4):467–72.

53. Kohli MR, Yamaguchi M, Setzer FC, et al. Spectrophotometric analysis of coro-nal tooth discoloration induced by various bioceramic cements and other end-odontic materials. J Endod 2015;41(11):1862–6.

54. Kang S-H, Shin Y-S, Lee H-S, et al. Color changes of teeth after treatment with various mineral trioxide aggregate–based materials: an ex vivo study. J Endod 2015;41(5):737–41.

55. Vallés M, Mercadé M, Duran-Sindreu F, et al. Influence of light and oxygen on the color stability of five calcium silicate–based materials. J Endod 2013; 39(4):525–8.

56. Machado J, Johnson JD, Paranjpe A. The effects of endosequence root repair material on differentiation of dental pulp cells. J Endod 2016;42(1):101–5.

57. Lyngstadaas SP, Wohlfahrt JC, Brookes SJ, et al. Enamel matrix proteins; old molecules for new applications. Orthod Craniofac Res 2009;12(3):243–53.

58. Lyngstadaas SP, Lundberg E, Ekdahl H, et al. Autocrine growth factors in human periodontal ligament cells cultured on enamel matrix derivative. J Clin Periodon-tol 2001;28(2):181–8.

59. Al-Hezaimi K, Al-Tayar BA, BaJuaifer YS, et al. A hybrid approach to direct pulp capping by using emdogain with a capping material. J Endodontics 2011;37(5): 667–72.

60. Schlueter SR, Carnes DL, Cochran DL. In vitro effects of enamel matrix deriva-tive on microvascular cells. J Periodontol 2007;78(1):141–51.

61. Suzuki S, Nagano T, Yamakoshi Y, et al. Enamel matrix derivative gel stimulates signal transduction of BMP and TGF-{beta}. J Dent Res 2005;84(6):510–4.

62. Weishaupt P, Bernimoulin JP, Trackman P, et al. Stimulation of osteoblasts with Emdogain increases the expression of specific mineralization markers. Oral Surg Oral Med Oral Pathol Oral Radiol Endod 2008;106(2):304–8.

63. Nakamura Y, Hammarstrom L, Lundberg E, et al. Enamel matrix derivative promotes reparative processes in the dental pulp. Adv Dent Res 2001;15:105–7.
64. Igarashi R, Sahara T, Shimizu-Ishiura M, et al. Porcine enamel matrix derivative enhances the formation of reparative dentine and dentine bridges during wound healing of amputated rat molars. J Electron Microsc (Tokyo) 2003;52(2):227–36.
65. Kiatwateeratana T, Kintarak S, Piwat S, et al. Partial pulpotomy on caries-free teeth using enamel matrix derivative or calcium hydroxide: a randomized controlled trial. Int Endod J 2009;42(7):584–92.
66. Olsson H, Davies JR, Holst KE, et al. Dental pulp capping: effect of Emdogain Gel on experimentally exposed human pulps. Int Endod J 2005;38(3):186–94.
67. Garrocho-Rangel A, Flores H, Silva-Herzog D, et al. Efficacy of EMD versus calcium hydroxide in direct pulp capping of primary molars: a randomized controlled clinical trial. Oral Surg Oral Med Oral Pathol Oral Radiol Endod 2009;107(5):733–8.
68. Qureshi A, E S, Nandakumar, Pratapkumar, et al. Recent advances in pulp capping materials: an overview. J Clin Diagn Res 2014;8(1):316–21.
69. Goldberg M. Pulp healing and regeneration: more questions than answers. Adv Dent Res 2011;23(3):270–4.
70. Arnett TR. Extracellular pH regulates bone cell function. J Nutr 2008;138(2):415S–8S.
71. Kohn DH, Sarmadi M, Helman JI, et al. Effects of pH on human bone marrow stromal cells in vitro: implications for tissue engineering of bone. J Biomed Mater Res 2002;60(2):292–9.
72. Brandao-Burch A, Utting JC, Orriss IR, et al. Acidosis inhibits bone formation by osteoblasts in vitro by preventing mineralization. Calcif Tissue Int 2005;77(3):167–74.
73. Golu EE, Boesze-Battaglia K. The role of alkaline phosphatase in mineralization. Curr Opin Orthop 2007;18:444–8.
74. Carrotte P. Endodontics: Part 9. Calcium hydroxide, root resorption, endo-perio lesions. Br Dent J 2004;197(12):735–43.
75. Staehle HJ, Pioch T, Hoppe W. The alkalizing properties of calcium hydroxide compounds. Endod Dent Traumatol 1989;5(3):147–52.
76. Glass RL, Zander HA. Pulp healing. J Dent Res 1949;28(2):97–107.
77. Tanomaru-Filho M, Chaves Faleiros FB, Sacaki JN, et al. Evaluation of pH and calcium ion release of root-end filling materials containing calcium hydroxide or mineral trioxide aggregate. J Endod 2009;35(10):1418–21.
78. Fridland M, Rosado R. MTA solubility: a long term study. J Endod 2005;31(5):376–9.
79. Fridland M, Rosado R. Mineral trioxide aggregate (MTA) solubility and porosity with different water-to-powder ratios. J Endod 2003;29(12):814–7.
80. Monfoulet LE, Becquart P, Marchat D, et al. The pH in the microenvironment of human mesenchymal stem cells is a critical factor for optimal osteogenesis in tissue-engineered constructs. Tissue Eng Part A 2014;20(13–14):1827–40.
81. Fliefel R, Popov C, Troltzsch M, et al. Mesenchymal stem cell proliferation and mineralization but not osteogenic differentiation are strongly affected by extracellular pH. J Craniomaxillofac Surg 2016;44(6):715–24.
82. Mohammadi Z, Dummer PM. Properties and applications of calcium hydroxide in endodontics and dental traumatology. Int Endod J 2011;44(8):697–730.
83. Siqueira JF Jr, Lopes HP. Mechanisms of antimicrobial activity of calcium hydroxide: a critical review. Int Endod J 1999;32(5):361–9.

84. Khan AA, Sun X, Hargreaves KM. Effect of calcium hydroxide on proinflammatory cytokines and neuropeptides. J Endod 2008;34(11):1360–3.

85. Reyes-Carmona JF, Santos AR, Figueiredo CP, et al. In vivo host interactions with mineral trioxide aggregate and calcium hydroxide: inflammatory molecular signaling assessment. J Endod 2011;37(9):1225–35.

86. Natale LC, Rodrigues MC, Xavier TA, et al. Ion release and mechanical properties of calcium silicate and calcium hydroxide materials used for pulp capping. Int Endod J 2015;48(1):89–94.

87. Sciaky I, Pisanti S. Localization of calcium placed over amputated pulps in dogs' teeth. J Dent Res 1960;39:1128–32.

88. Apati A, Paszty K, Erdei Z, et al. Calcium signaling in pluripotent stem cells. Mol Cell Endocrinol 2012;353(1–2):57–67.

89. Tonelli FM, Santos AK, Gomes DA, et al. Stem cells and calcium signaling. Adv Exp Med Biol 2012;740:891–916.

90. Dvorak MM, Siddiqua A, Ward DT, et al. Physiological changes in extracellular calcium concentration directly control osteoblast function in the absence of calciotropic hormones. Proc Natl Acad Sci U S A 2004;101(14):5140–5.

91. Matsuoka H, Akiyama H, Okada Y, et al. In vitro analysis of the stimulation of bone formation by highly bioactive apatite- and wollastonite-containing glass-ceramic: released calcium ions promote osteogenic differentiation in osteoblastic ROS17/2.8 cells. J Biomed Mater Res 1999;47(2):176–88.

92. Cheng S, Wang W, Lin Z, et al. Effects of extracellular calcium on viability and osteogenic differentiation of bone marrow stromal cells in vitro. Hum Cell 2013;26(3):114–20.

93. Nakamura S, Matsumoto T, Sasaki J, et al. Effect of calcium ion concentrations on osteogenic differentiation and hematopoietic stem cell niche-related protein expression in osteoblasts. Tissue Eng Part A 2010;16(8):2467–73.

94. Ma S, Yang Y, Carnes DL, et al. Effects of dissolved calcium and phosphorous on osteoblast responses. J Oral Implantol 2005;31(2):61–7.

95. Barradas AM, Yuan H, van der Stok J, et al. The influence of genetic factors on the osteoinductive potential of calcium phosphate ceramics in mice. Biomaterials 2012;33(23):5696–705.

96. Coathup MJ, Samizadeh S, Fang YS, et al. The osteoinductivity of silicate-substituted calcium phosphate. J Bone Joint Surg Am 2011;93(23):2219–26.

97. Chan O, Coathup MJ, Nesbitt A, et al. The effects of microporosity on osteoinduction of calcium phosphate bone graft substitute biomaterials. Acta Biomater 2012;8(7):2788–94.

98. Yuan H, Fernandes H, Habibovic P, et al. Osteoinductive ceramics as a synthetic alternative to autologous bone grafting. Proc Natl Acad Sci U S A 2010; 107(31):13614–9.

99. Hoppe A, Guldal NS, Boccaccini AR. A review of the biological response to ionic dissolution products from bioactive glasses and glass-ceramics. Biomaterials 2011;32(11):2757–74.

100. Barradas AM, Monticone V, Hulsman M, et al. Molecular mechanisms of biomaterial-driven osteogenic differentiation in human mesenchymal stromal cells. Integr Biol (Camb) 2013;5(7):920–31.

101. Tada H, Nemoto E, Kanaya S, et al. Elevated extracellular calcium increases expression of bone morphogenetic protein-2 gene via a calcium channel and ERK pathway in human dental pulp cells. Biochem Biophys Res Commun 2010;394(4):1093–7.

102. Rashid F, Shiba H, Mizuno N, et al. The effect of extracellular calcium ion on gene expression of bone-related proteins in human pulp cells. J Endod 2003; 29(2):104–7.

103. Mizuno M, Banzai Y. Calcium ion release from calcium hydroxide stimulated fibronectin gene expression in dental pulp cells and the differentiation of dental pulp cells to mineralized tissue forming cells by fibronectin. Int Endod J 2008; 41(11):933–8.

104. Kanaya S, Nemoto E, Ebe Y, et al. Elevated extracellular calcium increases fibroblast growth factor-2 gene and protein expression levels via a cAMP/PKA dependent pathway in cementoblasts. Bone 2010;47(3):564–72.

105. Aguirre A, Gonzalez A, Planell JA, et al. Extracellular calcium modulates in vitro bone marrow-derived Flk-1+ CD34+ progenitor cell chemotaxis and differentiation through a calcium-sensing receptor. Biochem Biophys Res Commun 2010; 393(1):156–61.

106. Gonzalez-Vazquez A, Planell JA, Engel E. Extracellular calcium and CaSR drive osteoinduction in mesenchymal stromal cells. Acta Biomater 2014;10(6): 2824–33.

107. Kim YH, Kim JM, Kim SN, et al. p44/42 MAPK activation is necessary for receptor activator of nuclear factor-kappaB ligand induction by high extracellular calcium. Biochem Biophys Res Commun 2003;304(4):729–35.

108. Tu Q, Pi M, Karsenty G, et al. Rescue of the skeletal phenotype in CasR-deficient mice by transfer onto the Gcm2 null background. J Clin Invest 2003;111(7): 1029–37.

109. Pi M, Garner SC, Flannery P, et al. Sensing of extracellular cations in CasR-deficient osteoblasts. Evidence for a novel cation-sensing mechanism. J Biol Chem 2000;275(5):3256–63.

110. Koori K, Maeda H, Fujii S, et al. The roles of calcium-sensing receptor and calcium channel in osteogenic differentiation of undifferentiated periodontal ligament cells. Cell Tissue Res 2014;357(3):707–18.

111. Zamponi GW. Targeting voltage-gated calcium channels in neurological and psychiatric diseases. Nat Rev Drug Discov 2016;15(1):19–34.

112. Wen L, Wang Y, Wang H, et al. L-type calcium channels play a crucial role in the proliferation and osteogenic differentiation of bone marrow mesenchymal stem cells. Biochem Biophys Res Commun 2012;424(3):439–45.

113. Bergh JJ, Shao Y, Puente E, et al. Osteoblast Ca(2+) permeability and voltage-sensitive Ca(2+) channel expression is temporally regulated by 1,25-dihydroxyvitamin D(3). Am J Physiol Cell Physiol 2006;290(3):C822–31.

114. Shin MK, Kim MK, Bae YS, et al. A novel collagen-binding peptide promotes osteogenic differentiation via Ca2+/calmodulin-dependent protein kinase II/ERK/AP-1 signaling pathway in human bone marrow-derived mesenchymal stem cells. Cell Signal 2008;20(4):613–24.

115. Barradas AM, Fernandes HA, Groen N, et al. A calcium-induced signaling cascade leading to osteogenic differentiation of human bone marrow-derived mesenchymal stromal cells. Biomaterials 2012;33(11):3205–15.

116. Ju Y, Ge J, Ren X, et al. Ca1.2 of L-type calcium channel is a key factor for the differentiation of dental pulp stem cells. J Endod 2015;41(7):1048–55.

117. Prakriya M, Feske S, Gwack Y, et al. Orai1 is an essential pore subunit of the CRAC channel. Nature 2006;443(7108):230–3.

118. Feske S, Gwack Y, Prakriya M, et al. A mutation in Orai1 causes immune deficiency by abrogating CRAC channel function. Nature 2006;441(7090):179–85.

119. Lee SH, Park Y, Song M, et al. Orai1 mediates osteogenic differentiation via BMP signaling pathway in bone marrow mesenchymal stem cells. Biochem Biophys Res Commun 2016;473(4):1309–14.

120. Robinson LJ, Mancarella S, Songsawad D, et al. Gene disruption of the calcium channel Orai1 results in inhibition of osteoclast and osteoblast differentiation and impairs skeletal development. Lab Invest 2012;92(7):1071–83.

121. Hwang SY, Foley J, Numaga-Tomita T, et al. Deletion of Orai1 alters expression of multiple genes during osteoclast and osteoblast maturation. Cell Calcium 2012;52(6):488–500.

122. Sohn S, Park Y, Srikanth S, et al. The Role of ORAI1 in the odontogenic differentiation of human dental pulp stem cells. J Dent Res 2015;94(11):1560–7.

123. Koliniotou-Koumpia E, Tziafas D. Pulpal responses following direct pulp capping of healthy dog teeth with dentine adhesive systems. J Dent 2005; 33(8):639–47.

124. Tarim B, Hafez AA, Cox CF. Pulpal response to a resin-modified glass-ionomer material on nonexposed and exposed monkey pulps. Quintessence Int 1998; 29(8):535–42.

125. Tziafa C, Koliniotou-Koumpia E, Papadimitriou S, et al. Dentinogenic responses after direct pulp capping of miniature swine teeth with Biodentine. J Endod 2014;40(12):1967–71.

126. Saito K, Nakatomi M, Ida-Yonemochi H, et al. Osteopontin is essential for type I collagen secretion in reparative dentin. J Dent Res 2016;95(9):1034–41.

127. Hunter DJ, Bardet C, Mouraret S, et al. Wnt acts as a pro-survival signal to enhance dentin regeneration. J Bone Miner Res 2015;30(7):1150–9.

# Regenerative Endodontic Procedures: Clinical Outcomes

Anibal Diogenes, DDS, MS, PhD*, Nikita B. Ruparel, MS, DDS, PhD

## KEYWORDS

- Revascularization • Regenerative endodontics • Immature teeth
- Root development • Revitalization

## KEY POINTS

- Regenerative endodontic procedures (REPs) are stem cell–based procedures.
- Translational science has been crucial for the development of disinfection protocols that also foster stem cell survival and differentiation.
- Currently used REPs achieve both primary and secondary outcomes, healing of apical periodontitis and root development, respectively. However, prognostic factors that influence these outcomes remain largely unknown.
- Reestablishment of positive responses seen in vitality testing suggests directional targeting of apical neurons into the newly formed tissue.
- Current evidence suggests that REPs promote guided-endodontic repair (GER) as opposed to "true regeneration" of a pulp-dentin complex indistinguishable from the native pulp.

The field of regenerative endodontics has dramatically evolved in the past decade. The initial case report of a revascularization in 2001,[1] followed by another report in 2004,[2] captured the attention of endodontists worldwide. In addition to the resolution of apical periodontitis, there was evidence of unprecedented continued root development and reestablishment of vitality responses with these procedures. For the first time, successful clinical outcomes in teeth diagnosed with pulp necrosis were reported without the obturation of the root canal with an inert material (gutta-percha) or a bioceramic material (eg, mineral trioxide aggregate). This represented a departure from the classic philosophy that a root canal had to be sealed once debrided to achieve resolution of apical periodontitis and that reestablishment of physiologic pulp-like responses was possible. This truly represented a paradigm shift introducing endodontics to the fields of regenerative medicine and dentistry.[3] Suddenly, a significant

Disclosure: The authors deny any conflict of interest related to this work.
Department of Endodontics, University of Texas Health Science Center at San Antonio, 7703 Floyd Curl Drive, San Antonio, TX 78229, USA
* Corresponding author.
*E-mail address:* Diogenes@uthscsa.edu

body of basic science research related to dentinogenesis, tooth development, and mesenchymal stem cell biology was adopted by this emerging field and provided a foundation for further advancements and translation into clinical practice.

The goal of regenerative endodontics is the use of biologic-based procedures to arrest the disease process, preventing its recurrence while favoring the repair or replacement of damaged structures of the pulp-dentin complex. Therefore, regenerative endodontics includes both vital and nonvital pulp therapies. Although vital pulp therapies, such as direct and indirect pulp capping, and pulpotomy procedures aim to preserve and maintain pulpal health in teeth that have been exposed to trauma, caries, restorative procedures, and anatomic anomalies, nonvital therapies include procedures that aim to reestablish a new vital tissue to replace dental pulp lost to liquefaction necrosis following infection. Several terms have been coined for these procedures that include "revascularization,"[1] "revitalization,"[4,5] and "maturogenesis,"[6] among others. However, for the sake of this review, we focus on nonvital pulp therapies and address to these procedures collectively as regenerative endodontic procedures (REPs).

## THE CLINICAL PROBLEM

Tooth development is a complex and long process of postnatal organogenesis. A tooth may take an additional 3 years after eruption to complete its development seen as complete root maturation.[7] The developing dentition is at risk for pulpal inflammation and necrosis due to trauma, caries, and developmental dental anomalies, such as dens evaginatus.[8–11] Loss of an immature permanent tooth in young patients with mixed dentition can be devastating, leading to loss of function; altered maxillary and mandibular bone development; interferences with phonetics, breathing, and mastication; and, importantly, there is a severe detrimental psychosocial effect on young patients.[12,13] Moreover, implants are contraindicated in patients undergoing cranioskeletal development, as their use has been associated with interferences in normal orofacial growth.[14] These teeth have been traditionally treated with apexification procedures using either long-term calcium hydroxide treatment[15,16] or immediate placement of a mineral trioxide aggregate (MTA) apical plug.[17] Although these treatments often result in the resolution of signs and symptoms of pathosis, they provide little to no benefit for continued root development,[18] remaining with thin fragile dentinal walls increasing susceptibility to fractures and lower survival.[15,19] A study evaluating root fractures after apexification procedures in 885 luxated nonvital incisors clearly demonstrated that as low as 28% and as high as 77% of the teeth had cervical root fractures owing to the least amount of dentin present in this area.[15] Therefore, clinicians must make use of all means necessary to retain the natural dentition through childhood and adolescence years, and hopefully beyond the maturation stage. To attain this goal, both vital pulp and nonvital pulp regenerative therapies should be considered.

It is important to note that most published regenerative endodontic cases, but not all,[20] report treatment outcomes in immature teeth with an open apex.[11] The degree of root formation and tooth maturation can be broadly classified according to previously established criteria (**Fig. 1**).[7,21,22] The great majority of cases treated with REPs are of teeth in stages 2 through 5, which include teeth with at least half of the root formed but with an open "blunderbuss" apex, or teeth that have achieved maximum root elongation but lack thickening of the dentinal wall and present with an open apex. As mentioned previously, the use of REPs in endodontics is not exclusive to immature teeth, because there have been cases published reporting

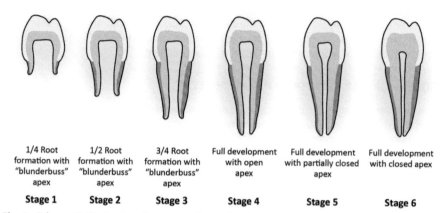

| 1/4 Root formation with "blunderbuss" apex | 1/2 Root formation with "blunderbuss" apex | 3/4 Root formation with "blunderbuss" apex | Full development with open apex | Full development with partially closed apex | Full development with closed apex |
|---|---|---|---|---|---|
| **Stage 1** | **Stage 2** | **Stage 3** | **Stage 4** | **Stage 5** | **Stage 6** |

**Fig. 1.** Schematic illustrating the stages of root development. Roots elongate while maintaining an open apex that at later stages narrows followed by thickening of the dentinal walls.

successful outcomes in teeth in stages 5 and 6 of maturation (mature fully formed teeth),[20,23] including a case series.[24]

The preferential use of REPs in immature teeth is largely based on observation from the trauma literature that immature teeth have greater potential for "self-revascularization" after severe trauma. In a study, replanted teeth after avulsion had significantly greater change of regaining pulp vitality responses if the apex demonstrated at least 1 mm in diameter on a periapical radiograph.[25] This observation is further supported by other studies showing that immature teeth had greater clinical success without the need for endodontic intervention than teeth that were further developed.[26–28] Although the process of tissue formation in regenerative endodontics greatly differs from the process of revascularization of an existing sterile pulp as seen in replantation, it equally relies on angiogenesis and the ingress of newly formed blood vessels through the apical opening.[29,30] Clinicians rely on the transfer of undifferentiated mesenchymal stem cells (MSCs) into the root canal system that is attained by evoked bleeding from the apical region, including possibly the apical papilla.[31] Although a recent study demonstrated that MSCs also can be transferred into canals of mature teeth in patients far into adulthood,[32] there is compelling evidence that proliferation,[33] differentiation,[34] and overall regenerative potential[35] of MSCs decrease with age. Further research is required to investigate whether these "aged MSCs," if transferred autologously into root canals, could lead to successful clinical outcomes similar to those observed in immature teeth. Also, it would be important to investigate whether "aged MSCs" could be rejuvenated clinically as demonstrated in some basic science investigations. The transition of regenerative procedures will require careful consideration, as the challenges to be overcome appear greater than in immature teeth and conventional endodontics in mature teeth has well documented excellent clinical outcomes.[36]

Interestingly, the effects of root development stage and apical diameter on clinical outcomes of REPs have never been established. A recent preclinical study found that vascularized tissue could be formed in teeth with an apical diameter of approximately 0.3 mm, which is similar to the apical diameter of most canals in fully mature roots.[37,38] Also, a clinical study demonstrated that without apical enlargement, MSCs could be transferred into root canals of mature teeth with evoked apical bleeding,[32] and successful outcomes have been reported for mature teeth treated with REPs in adults [20,23,24]. In summary, most REPs have been performed in immature teeth, but the minimum apical diameter for successful outcomes has not been established. Recent studies and a case report challenge the preconceived notion that an apical diameter greater than 1 mm is a requirement for desirable outcomes in REPs,[37] and that REPs should be limited only for immature teeth in young patients.

## ETIOLOGY OF PULP NECROSIS IN IMMATURE TEETH

Etiologies for a necrotic pulp range from trauma to caries to congenital anomalies. Trauma has been recognized as the primary etiology of pulpal necrosis in immature permanent teeth.[11] Up to 35% of children,[39] particularly between the ages of 7 and 15 years,[40,41] experience traumatic dental injuries when most permanent teeth are in incomplete stage of root development. Approximately one-half of teeth are likely to be diagnosed with pulpal necrosis,[42] with greater incidence occurring after severe injuries, such as intrusions and avulsions[27,43] and combination injuries.[44–46] Therefore, the high incidence of trauma-evoked pulpal necrosis reported in the patients included in case reports, and retrospective and prospective studies in regenerative endodontics is likely biased by the high incidence of these injuries. Moderate to severe trauma to the developing dentition can potentially damage the Hertwig epithelial root sheath (HERS), known to be crucial for formation and maturation of roots by directing the concerted proliferation and differentiation of MSCs.[47] A study that evaluated traumatized teeth treated with REPs reported that although most teeth demonstrated adequate healing of apical periodontitis, resolution of symptoms, and apical closure, there was unpredictable root development.[48] Perhaps this may be due to trauma being an etiology with varied severity (eg, intrusions vs luxations) and potential of damaging the HERS. Studies with larger cohorts are needed to evaluate prognostic factors related to continuation of root development following REPs.

The second most common etiology of pulp necrosis in immature teeth is the presence of either dens evaginatus or dens invaginatus (approximately 36% of cases treated with REPs).[9–11] Dens evaginatus is more common between these 2 dental anomalies, accounting for the etiology of approximately 33% of cases treated with REPs. It is seen on clinical and radiographic examination as an additional cusp, typically projecting into the occlusal table of a mandibular premolar (more common) or the facial or lingual surfaces of maxillary anterior teeth (less common). The incidence of dens evaginatus has been reported to affect up to 6% of the population, with greater incidence in certain ethnic groups.[49,50] Although the incidence of this dental anomaly is relatively rare, its presence often leads to rapid pulp necrosis once teeth affected are in functional occlusion, ensuring the enamel-dentinal tubercle and direct exposure of the pulp to the oral environment. The subsequent rapid manifestation of symptoms related to pulpitis and the infection encourage patients to seek immediate care. Perhaps, early intervention and the absence of trauma to apical structures results in typically observed good clinical outcomes in these cases. Nonetheless, studies comparing outcomes following REPs in teeth with different etiologies are needed to substantiate this observation.

## COMMON FEATURES OF REGENERATIVE ENDODONTIC PROCEDURES FOR THE TREATMENT OF IMMATURE TEETH WITH PULPAL NECROSIS

REPs in immature teeth with pulpal necrosis have 3 main components:

1. Disinfection
2. Recruitment of MSCs and establishment of a scaffold
3. Placement of a coronal barrier and restoration

## Disinfection

Eliminating microbial biofilm is of paramount importance in any endodontic procedure. However, in a REP, disinfection also sets the stage for a stem cell–conducive environment.[51] MSCs from the periapical tissues, such as the apical papilla and the periodontal ligament, are recruited into the root canal system and are thought to mediate the regenerative processes. Because a variety of factors affect stem cell survival and differentiation, it is crucial to pay close attention to the exogenous materials that are introduced into the canal system for disinfection as well as preexisting biofilms.

The current American Association of Endodontist (AAE) and European Endodontic Society (ESE)[52] guidelines recommend minimal to no instrumentation of the canal systems to preserve remaining dentin; REPs therefore rely entirely on chemical disinfection for elimination of microbial biofilm and their by-products. The commonly used chemical disinfectants include irrigants, such as sodium hypochlorite (NaOCl), EDTA, and chlorhexidine (CHX), and intracanal medicaments, such as triple antibiotic paste (TAP), double antibiotic paste (DAP), or calcium hydroxide (Ca[OH]$_2$), among others.[11,51,53] Extensive research on the effects of each of the commonly used irrigants and intracanal medicaments on the survival and fate of stem cell have shown that highly concentrated solutions of NaOCl are severely detrimental to the survival and differentiation capacity of stem cells.[54–56] Hugely beneficial effects of EDTA have been seen when used as a final irrigant before recruitment of stem cells from periapical tissues.[57] These effects are primarily attributed to the EDTA-induced release of growth factors from dentin that are capable of mediating stem cell chemotaxis and differentiation, angiogenesis, and neurogenesis (**Fig. 2**).[58–60] Similar to irrigants, such as full-strength NaOCl, undiluted TAP and DAP,[61,62] among other medicaments, have shown significant detrimental effects on stem cell survival, whereas full-strength Ca(OH)$_2$ or 1 mg/mL TAP/DAP are optimal for stem cell survival.[61,62] Additionally, recent studies also demonstrate adequate bactericidal effects and substantive effects of a 1 mg/mL concentration of DAP and that this residual effect has been demonstrated to significantly reduce *Enterococcus faecalis* biofilm.[63–65]

Therefore, to accomplish a conducive microenvironment for regeneration while achieving maximal bactericidal efficacy, 1.5% NaOCl followed by 17% EDTA and using either 1 mg/mL TAP or DAP or Ca(OH)$_2$ is recommended.

## Recruitment of Apical Mesenchymal Stem Cells and Establishment of a Scaffold

The initial use of evoked bleeding in REPs (ie, revascularization) was based on the seminal work by Dr Nyggard-Ostby[66] 50 years before the first contemporary case report that investigated the role of a blood clot in apical healing. It was not until 2011 that a clinical study demonstrated that the action of lacerating the apical tissues delivered substantial concentrations of MSCs into root canals in patients.[31] A suitable 3-dimensional (3-D) matrix allows for appropriate organization of stem cells and allows for cell-cell interactions during a regenerative process. Therefore, the formation of a fibrin network in the blood clot acts as a scaffold for cells grown in a 3-D matrix. However, some published cases indicate obtaining an adequate blood clot as an unpredictable outcome. Thus, other scaffolding matrices, such platelet rich plasma (PRP),[4] platelet rich fibrin (PRF),[67] and injectable scaffold impregnated with fibroblast-derived growth factor,[68] have been used and demonstrate comparable success to a blood clot.

## Placement of a Coronal Barrier and Restoration

Another important step seen in most published cases is the coronal placement of a bioactive "coronal plug" using promineralizing dental materials, such as MTA or

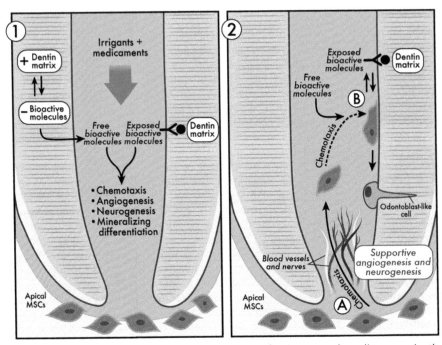

**Fig. 2.** Schematic illustrating the potential actions of irrigants and medicaments in the release and/or exposure of bioactive molecules sequestered in dentin and their influences on regenerative events, including chemotaxis, odontoblastlike cell differentiation, mineralization, angiogenesis, and neurogenesis. (*From* Smith AJ, Duncan HF, Diogenes A, et al. Exploiting the bioactive properties of the dentin-pulp complex in regenerative endodontics. J Endod 2016;42(1):50; with permission.)

Biodentine, among other bioceramic materials.[53] These materials have been shown to promote the differentiation of MSCs into an odontoblastlike phenotype while allowing for enhanced proliferation of MSCs.[69–72] Importantly, they provide a "safe-zone" barrier to the restorative material used to seal the pulp chamber that is typically noxious to stem cell survival and differentiation. Interestingly, there have been case reports of REPs performed without the use of these materials with acceptable clinical outcomes.[53] Therefore, the role of the bioactive coronal plug in promoting the proliferation and differentiation of MSCs throughout the length of the canal is not fully understood. Nonetheless, in certain cases a calcific barrier can be seen immediately underneath the material (**Fig. 3**), suggesting that these materials are capable of inducing differentiation of stem cells in vivo, potentially leading to the formation of a biological coronal seal.

Coronal discoloration related to the placement of an MTA coronal barrier has been reported even when the white form of the material is used.[73–77] This undesirable result can be minimized by occluding the coronal dentinal tubules with a dental adhesive,[78] or largely prevented by the use of other bioceramic materials, such as Biodentine (Septodont, France) and Endosequence (Brasseler, Switzerland) in esthetic zones.[79–82] In addition to their improved color stability and reduced staining potential than MTA, these materials have been shown to also promote proliferation and odontogenic differentiation of MSCs.[69,83] Also, they can potentially be placed above the cementoenamel junction due to their handling characteristics and reduced risk of

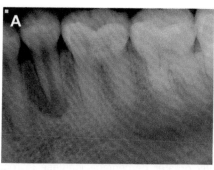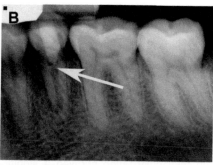

**Fig. 3.** A 27-year-old woman patient presented with sinus tract associated with tooth #20 diagnosed with dens evaginatus and pulpal necrosis and chronic apical abscess. The patient reported discomfort on the tooth for several years. A large radiolucency associated with the open apex of the immature root with thin dentinal walls was observed in the preoperative radiograph (*A*). The tooth was treated with a REP following AAE-recommended guidelines. The patient presented asymptomatic and with resolution of the sinus tract 30 days after the first visit for completion of the treatment. At the 2-year follow-up appointment, the patient was still asymptomatic, and the tooth responded repeatedly to electric pulp testing. In addition, there was evidence of complete resolution of the radiolucency, thickening of the dentinal walls, and the presence of a mineralized bridge immediately below the MTA layer on the postoperative radiograph (*yellow arrow, B*). (*Courtesy of* Dr Blake Ishikawa, DDS, University of Texas Health Science Center at San Antonio, San Antonio, TX, USA.)

tooth discoloration. Coronal placement of these bioactive materials is a desirable advantage, because cervical hard tissue deposition can potentially increase resistance to fracture and long-term tooth survival.

## CLINICAL OUTCOMES

REPs as a new treatment modality must be objectively compared with the longer established, more traditional endodontic treatment procedures for immature teeth, namely apexification procedures.[11,84]

## PRIMARY TREATMENT GOAL

The primary concern for a practicing clinician must be to promote healing of the diseased tissues, prevention of disease relapse, and patient well-being (patient-centered outcomes).[85] Thus, the primary therapeutic goal of REPs must be resolution of apical periodontitis while promoting the survival and function of the tooth. In 2012, a retrospective study aimed to directly compare the clinical outcomes of apexification and REPs.[19] This study was the first to compare both procedures performed under standardized protocols, and included apexification procedures performed with the use of MTA as an apical plug or the long-term use of calcium hydroxide.[19] Resolution of the disease process (no pain, swelling, or sinus tracts) was found in 100% of the REPs, 95% of the MTA apexification, and 77% of calcium hydroxide apexification cases. On the other hand, another retrospective study that did not include standardization of treatment protocols found REPs to promote healing in 79% of patients treated, whereas apexification procedures promoted healing in 100% of the patients; this difference was found not to be significant.[86] In a prospective study, both MTA apexification and REPs were found to promote healing in 100% of all patients.[68] Further evidence of successful outcomes can be found in case series and retrospective patient cohort studies. Despite significant variations in etiology and inclusion and exclusion criteria, these studies demonstrate that on average both procedures successfully resolve the signs and symptoms of the disease in approximately 90% of patients.

## SECONDARY TREATMENT GOAL

A secondary therapeutic goal of REPs is continued root development. In 2009 a retrospective study was the first to use an objective dependent measure of root development to compare radiographic root development between apexification procedures (n = 40) and REPs (n = 48).[18] These findings have been confirmed by Jeeruphan and colleagues[19] using a similar quantitative technique, reporting that teeth treated with revascularization showed a significantly greater percentage increase in root length (14.9%) compared with teeth treated by either MTA apexification (6.1%) or calcium hydroxide apexification (0.4%). They also reported that the revascularization protocol produced significantly greater percentage increases in root width (28.2%) compared with teeth treated by either MTA apexification (0.0%) or calcium hydroxide apexification (1.52%).[19] Further evidence of continued root development following REPs can be found in a prospective randomized clinical trial that compared 2 different protocols of REPs with MTA apexification procedures.[68] Regenerative procedures promoted an average increase of 12% in root thickness and a 50% decrease in apical diameter (apical closure), whereas apexification procedures demonstrated no change during the 18-month observation period.[68] Interestingly, a recent retrospective study reported that degree of root development was highly varied and unpredictable.[86] This discrepancy is likely due to the greater number of included cases with trauma as the etiology for pulpal necrosis, and the relatively small sample size.

Collectively, the studies using quantitative analysis have provided evidence that REPs promote increase in radiographic root development in most cases, but not all. The factors that influence this lack of response in certain cases are largely unknown, but could include the persistence of bacterial biofilms or antigens, the nature of the etiology, delay in treatment, and the impact of disinfection agents on the creation of a microenvironment conducive to regeneration.

Root development is considered a secondary goal of REPs because it is expected to increase resistance to fracture and tooth survival. In a retrospective study including more than 1.4 million patients, conventional root canal therapy was found to promote the 8-year survival in 97% of the cases.[36] Unfortunately, far less is known regarding the long-term survival of immature teeth treated with either apexification or REPs. A retrospective study compared the survival of teeth treated with either REPs or apexification procedures with calcium hydroxide or placement of an MTA apical plug.[19] The survival of teeth treated with REPs (100% of teeth survived) during the follow-up period of the study (18 months) was significantly greater than that of teeth treated with calcium hydroxide (77%), but not different from teeth treated with an MTA apical plug (95%). These findings are in agreement with previous reports that prolonged use of calcium hydroxide can significantly weaken teeth, increasing their susceptibility to fracture.[15,87] In summary, REPs have been shown to arrest the disease process and allow for retention of teeth with otherwise very poor prognosis in patients still undergoing cranioskeletal development. Factors affecting the long-term survival of these teeth require further investigation with studies using appropriate sample sizes and follow-up.

## TERTIARY TREATMENT GOAL

Return of pulp vitality has been reported in approximately 50% of all published REPs.[11] The presence of functional nociceptors following REPs suggests that apically positioned free nerve endings of primary afferents are guided into the canal by specific chemical signals. Perhaps this process of axonal guidance is similar to the targeting of axons from trigeminal sensory neurons that accumulate forming a plexus beneath the tooth organ and dental follicle, but do not enter the apical papilla until late bell stage and during the eruption process. This process is guided by a balance between neuro-attractant and neuro-repelling molecules.[88,89] The undifferentiated cells of the apical papilla or stem cells of the apical papilla during tooth development express these molecules at the earliest stages of tooth development, and have been implicated and the primary cell type guiding axonal navigation and targeting into the developing tooth.[89] Interestingly, the same cells (ie, stem cells of the apical papilla SCAP) are believed to be a prominent cell type in REPs in immature teeth.[11,90]

A recent study sought to investigate whether postdevelopment SCAP could direct trigeminal neuronal targeting and innervation.[91] It demonstrated that SCAP harvested from an erupted third molar mediated robust axonal growth and targeting through the release of brain-derived neurotrophic factor (BDNF)[91] Interestingly, complete pulpal regeneration, including innervation, was achieved in dogs with the use of autologous transplantation of DPSCs.[92] Similarly, these cells were found to express high levels of BDNF compared with adipose and bone marrow MSCs.[93] Collectively, these findings support the hypothesis that MSCs transferred into the root canal space during REPs are likely important in the recruitment of apical primary afferent fibers through a specific mechanism of postnatal axonal targeting. The exact mechanism by which these newly recruited neurons respond to the different stimuli used in vitality testing warrants further investigation. Nonetheless, the presence of innervation suggests the presence of a vital tissue that is immune-competent due to the intimate association of innervation with blood vessels and the immune system. It also suggests the recovery of nociception that is crucial for the detection of actual or potential injury to the tooth organ.

## REPAIR OR REGENERATION

There is considerable debate on the use of the term "regeneration" because there is compelling evidence from histologic studies that the newly formed tissue following current forms of REPs does not resemble the lost pulp-dentin complex.[94–96] Instead, these procedures allow for repair to take place with evident recovery of certain physiologic responses.[97] To date, even in sophisticated animal models, tissues formed closely resemble the native dental pulp but true odontoblasts are missing; instead, mineralizing cells called "odontoblastlike cells" are formed.[92,98] Thus, the definition of regeneration depends largely on individual differences of its definition and the methodology to evaluate its presence, and appears to fall short when more advanced molecular techniques are used. Perhaps a more conservative term to be used to describe this procedure as it currently stands is guided-endodontic repair (GER); however, a repaired tissue that promotes resolution of the disease and reestablishment of some or all the original tissue functions should be an acceptable goal. From a patient-centered outcome perspective, shortcomings in histologic regeneration do not represent a failure.[85] Also, from a clinician perspective, a treated tooth that is asymptomatic, without any signs of disease and is functional should be considered a success.[85] From a scientific perspective, the lack of control of the tissues formed represents the status of the current procedures. The primary focus should be on how to achieve predictable root development in patients with the goal of improving clinical outcomes. Significantly more research and development is necessary to reach more sophisticated form of REPs that allow better control of the tissues formed. However, current forms of REPs, despite their shortcomings, have demonstrated clinically relevant acceptable outcomes and represent a treatment alternative to teeth with an otherwise poor prognosis.

It is important to highlight that the dental pulp capacity of repair seen in direct and indirect pulp-capping procedures, and in successful self-revascularization cases after trauma is absent once the pulp completely succumbs to infection or trauma. In these cases, clinicians using the knowledge gained in the field of regenerative endodontics are able to perform GER by directing the formation of a reparative tissue displaying once lost physiologic functions, such as vascularity, nociception, and mineral tissue deposition. This is achieved by the clinical application of tissue engineering principles with the goal of achieving maximum disinfection while creating the most conducive environment for stem cells to direct the repair and regeneration of the target tissue. Future developments will likely allow clinicians to place elaborate scaffolds with chemotactic agents to promote the repopulation of the root canal system in a spatial and temporal organized fashion, perhaps better achieving the desired histologic evidence of "regeneration." The pursuit of knowledge and development through translational science is promoting marked advances in the relatively young field of regenerative endodontics while promoting the retention of compromised immature teeth.

## REFERENCES

1. Iwaya SI, Ikawa M, Kubota M. Revascularization of an immature permanent tooth with apical periodontitis and sinus tract. Dent Traumatol 2001;17(4):185–7.
2. Banchs F, Trope M. Revascularization of immature permanent teeth with apical periodontitis: new treatment protocol? J Endod 2004;30(4):196–200.
3. Murray PE, Garcia-Godoy F, Hargreaves KM. Regenerative endodontics: a review of current status and a call for action. J Endod 2007;33(4):377–90.
4. Torabinejad M, Turman M. Revitalization of tooth with necrotic pulp and open apex by using platelet-rich plasma: a case report. J Endod 2011;37(2):265–8.
5. Wang X, Thibodeau B, Trope M, et al. Histologic characterization of regenerated tissues in canal space after the revitalization/revascularization procedure of immature dog teeth with apical periodontitis. J Endod 2010;36(1):56–63.
6. Aggarwal V, Miglani S, Singla M. Conventional apexification and revascularization induced maturogenesis of two non-vital, immature teeth in same patient: 24 months follow up of a case. J Conserv Dent 2012;15(1):68–72.
7. Moorrees CF, Fanning EA, Hunt EE Jr. Age variation of formation stages for ten permanent teeth. J Dent Res 1963;42:1490–502.
8. Cortes MI, Marcenes W, Sheiham A. Prevalence and correlates of traumatic injuries to the permanent teeth of schoolchildren aged 9-14 years in Belo Horizonte, Brazil. Dent Traumatol 2001;17(1):22–6.
9. Oehlers FA, Lee KW, Lee EC. Dens evaginatus (evaginated odontome). Its structure and responses to external stimuli. Dent Pract Dent Rec 1967;17(7):239–44.
10. Levitan ME, Himel VT. Dens evaginatus: literature review, pathophysiology, and comprehensive treatment regimen. J Endod 2006;32(1):1–9.
11. Diogenes A, Henry MA, Teixeira FB, et al. An update on clinical regenerative endodontics. Endod Top 2013;28(1):2–23.
12. Judd PL, Casas MJ. Psychosocial perceptions of premature tooth loss in children. Ont Dent 1995;72(8):16–8, 20, 22-13.
13. Thelen DS, Trovik TA, Bardsen A. Impact of traumatic dental injuries with unmet treatment need on daily life among Albanian adolescents: a case-control study. Dent Traumatol 2011;27(2):88–94.

14. Heij DG, Opdebeeck H, van Steenberghe D, et al. Facial development, continuous tooth eruption, and mesial drift as compromising factors for implant placement. Int J Oral Maxillofac Implants 2006;21(6):867–78.

15. Cvek M. Prognosis of luxated non-vital maxillary incisors treated with calcium hydroxide and filled with gutta-percha. A retrospective clinical study. Endod Dent Traumatol 1992;8(2):45–55.

16. Cvek M. Treatment of non-vital permanent incisors with calcium hydroxide. I. Follow-up of periapical repair and apical closure of immature roots. Odontol Revy 1972;23(1):27–44.

17. Witherspoon DE, Ham K. One-visit apexification: technique for inducing root-end barrier formation in apical closures. Pract Proced Aesthet Dent 2001;13(6): 455–60 [quiz: 462].

18. Bose R, Nummikoski P, Hargreaves K. A retrospective evaluation of radiographic outcomes in immature teeth with necrotic root canal systems treated with regenerative endodontic procedures. J Endod 2009;35(10):1343–9.

19. Jeeruphan T, Jantarat J, Yanpiset K, et al. Mahidol study 1: comparison of radiographic and survival outcomes of immature teeth treated with either regenerative endodontic or apexification methods: a retrospective study. J Endod 2012; 38(10):1330–6.

20. Paryani K, Kim SG. Regenerative endodontic treatment of permanent teeth after completion of root development: a report of 2 cases. J Endod 2013;39(7):929–34.

21. Moorrees CF, Gron AM, Lebret LM, et al. Growth studies of the dentition: a review. Am J Orthod 1969;55(6):600–16.

22. Moorrees CF, Kent RL Jr. Interrelations in the timing of root formation and tooth emergence. Proc Finn Dent Soc 1981;77(1–3):113–7.

23. Saoud TM, Sigurdsson A, Rosenberg PA, et al. Treatment of a large cystlike inflammatory periapical lesion associated with mature necrotic teeth using regenerative endodontic therapy. J Endod 2014;40(12):2081–6.

24. Saoud TM, Martin G, Chen YH, et al. Treatment of mature permanent teeth with necrotic pulps and apical periodontitis using regenerative endodontic procedures: a case series. J Endod 2016;42(1):57–65.

25. Kling M, Cvek M, Mejare I. Rate and predictability of pulp revascularization in therapeutically reimplanted permanent incisors. Endod Dent Traumatol 1986; 2(3):83–9.

26. Andreasen JO, Borum MK, Andreasen FM. Replantation of 400 avulsed permanent incisors. 3. Factors related to root growth. Endod Dent Traumatol 1995; 11(2):69–75.

27. Andreasen JO, Borum MK, Jacobsen HL, et al. Replantation of 400 avulsed permanent incisors. 2. Factors related to pulpal healing. Endod Dent Traumatol 1995; 11(2):59–68.

28. Andreasen JO, Hjorting-Hansen E. Replantation of teeth. I. Radiographic and clinical study of 110 human teeth replanted after accidental loss. Acta Odontol Scand 1966;24(3):263–86.

29. Skoglund A. Vascular changes in replanted and autotransplanted apicoectomized mature teeth of dogs. Int J Oral Surg 1981;10(2):100–10.

30. Skoglund A, Tronstad L, Wallenius K. A microangiographic study of vascular changes in replanted and autotransplanted teeth of young dogs. Oral Surg Oral Med Oral Pathol 1978;45(1):17–28.

31. Lovelace TW, Henry MA, Hargreaves KM, et al. Evaluation of the delivery of mesenchymal stem cells into the root canal space of necrotic immature teeth after clinical regenerative endodontic procedure. J Endod 2011;37(2):133–8.

32. Chrepa V, Henry MA, Daniel BJ, et al. Delivery of apical mesenchymal stem cells into root canals of mature teeth. J Dent Res 2015;94(12):1653–9.

33. Choumerianou DM, Martimianaki G, Stiakaki E, et al. Comparative study of stemness characteristics of mesenchymal cells from bone marrow of children and adults. Cytotherapy 2010;12(7):881–7.

34. Zhou S, Greenberger JS, Epperly MW, et al. Age-related intrinsic changes in human bone-marrow-derived mesenchymal stem cells and their differentiation to osteoblasts. Aging Cell 2008;7(3):335–43.

35. Iohara K, Murakami M, Nakata K, et al. Age-dependent decline in dental pulp regeneration after pulpectomy in dogs. Exp Gerontol 2014;52:39–45.

36. Salehrabi R, Rotstein I. Endodontic treatment outcomes in a large patient population in the USA: an epidemiological study. J Endod 2004;30(12):846–50.

37. Laureys WG, Cuvelier CA, Dermaut LR, et al. The critical apical diameter to obtain regeneration of the pulp tissue after tooth transplantation, replantation, or regenerative endodontic treatment. J Endod 2013;39(6):759–63.

38. Green EN. Microscopic investigation of root canal diameters. J Am Dent Assoc 1958;57(5):636–44.

39. Andreasen JO, Ravn JJ. Epidemiology of traumatic dental injuries to primary and permanent teeth in a Danish population sample. Int J Oral Surg 1972;1(5):235–9.

40. Forsberg CM, Tedestam G. Traumatic injuries to teeth in Swedish children living in an urban area. Swed Dent J 1990;14(3):115–22.

41. Forsberg CM, Tedestam G. Etiological and predisposing factors related to traumatic injuries to permanent teeth. Swed Dent J 1993;17(5):183–90.

42. Robertson A, Andreasen FM, Bergenholtz G, et al. Incidence of pulp necrosis subsequent to pulp canal obliteration from trauma of permanent incisors. J Endod 1996;22(10):557–60.

43. Andreasen JO, Bakland LK, Andreasen FM. Traumatic intrusion of permanent teeth. Part 3. A clinical study of the effect of treatment variables such as treatment delay, method of repositioning, type of splint, length of splinting and antibiotics on 140 teeth. Dent Traumatol 2006;22(2):99–111.

44. Lauridsen E, Hermann NV, Gerds TA, et al. Combination injuries 3. The risk of pulp necrosis in permanent teeth with extrusion or lateral luxation and concomitant crown fractures without pulp exposure. Dent Traumatol 2012;28(5):379–85.

45. Lauridsen E, Hermann NV, Gerds TA, et al. Combination injuries 1. The risk of pulp necrosis in permanent teeth with concussion injuries and concomitant crown fractures. Dent Traumatol 2012;28(5):364–70.

46. Lauridsen E, Hermann NV, Gerds TA, et al. Combination injuries 2. The risk of pulp necrosis in permanent teeth with subluxation injuries and concomitant crown fractures. Dent Traumatol 2012;28(5):371–8.

47. Xu L, Tang L, Jin F, et al. The apical region of developing tooth root constitutes a complex and maintains the ability to generate root and periodontium-like tissues. J Periodont Res 2009;44(2):275–82.

48. Saoud TM, Zaazou A, Nabil A, et al. Clinical and radiographic outcomes of traumatized immature permanent necrotic teeth after revascularization/revitalization therapy. J Endod 2014;40(12):1946–52.

49. Yip WK. The prevalence of dens evaginatus. Oral Surg Oral Med Oral Pathol 1974;38(1):80–7.

50. Temilola DO, Folayan MO, Fatusi O, et al. The prevalence, pattern and clinical presentation of developmental dental hard-tissue anomalies in children with primary and mix dentition from Ile-Ife, Nigeria. BMC Oral Health 2014;14:125.

51. Diogenes AR, Ruparel NB, Teixeira FB, et al. Translational science in disinfection for regenerative endodontics. J Endod 2014;40(4 Suppl):S52–7.
52. Galler KM, Krastl G, Simon S, et al. European Society of Endodontology Position Statement: revitalisation procedures. Int Endod J 2016;49(8):717–23.
53. Kontakiotis EG, Filippatos CG, Tzanetakis GN, et al. Regenerative endodontic therapy: a data analysis of clinical protocols. J Endod 2015;41(2):146–54.
54. Galler KM, Buchalla W, Hiller KA, et al. Influence of root canal disinfectants on growth factor release from dentin. J Endod 2015;41(3):363–8.
55. Trevino EG, Patwardhan AN, Henry MA, et al. Effect of irrigants on the survival of human stem cells of the apical papilla in a platelet-rich plasma scaffold in human root tips. J Endod 2011;37(8):1109–15.
56. Martin DE, Henry MA, Almeida JFA, et al. Effect of sodium hypochlorite on the odontoblastic phenotype differentiation of SCAP in cultured organotype human roots. J Endod 2012;38(3):e26.
57. Avivi-Arber L, Martin R, Lee JC, et al. Face sensorimotor cortex and its neuroplasticity related to orofacial sensorimotor functions. Arch Oral Biol 2011;56(12): 1440–65.
58. Galler KM, D'Souza RN, Federlin M, et al. Dentin conditioning codetermines cell fate in regenerative endodontics. J Endod 2011;37(11):1536–41.
59. Casagrande L, Demarco FF, Zhang Z, et al. Dentin-derived BMP-2 and odontoblast differentiation. J Dent Res 2010;89(6):603–8.
60. Smith AJ, Duncan HF, Diogenes A, et al. Exploiting the bioactive properties of the dentin-pulp complex in regenerative endodontics. J Endod 2016;42(1):47–56.
61. Ruparel NB, Teixeira FB, Ferraz CC, et al. Direct effect of intracanal medicaments on survival of stem cells of the apical papilla. J Endod 2012;38(10):1372–5.
62. Althumairy RI, Teixeira FB, Diogenes A. Effect of dentin conditioning with intracanal medicaments on survival of stem cells of apical papilla. J Endod 2014;40(4): 521–5.
63. Sabrah AH, Yassen GH, Gregory RL. Effectiveness of antibiotic medicaments against biofilm formation of *Enterococcus faecalis* and *Porphyromonas gingivalis*. J Endod 2013;39(11):1385–9.
64. Sabrah AH, Yassen GH, Liu WC, et al. The effect of diluted triple and double antibiotic pastes on dental pulp stem cells and established *Enterococcus faecalis* biofilm. Clin Oral Investig 2015;19(8):2059–66.
65. Sabrah AH, Yassen GH, Spolnik KJ, et al. Evaluation of residual antibacterial effect of human radicular dentin treated with triple and double antibiotic pastes. J Endod 2015;41(7):1081–4.
66. Ostby BN. The role of the blood clot in endodontic therapy. An experimental histologic study. Acta Odontol Scand 1961;19:324–53.
67. Shivashankar VY, Johns DA, Vidyanath S, et al. Platelet rich fibrin in the revitalization of tooth with necrotic pulp and open apex. J Conserv Dent 2012;15(4):395–8.
68. Nagy MM, Tawfik HE, Hashem AA, et al. Regenerative potential of immature permanent teeth with necrotic pulps after different regenerative protocols. J Endod 2014;40(2):192–8.
69. Zanini M, Sautier JM, Berdal A, et al. Biodentine induces immortalized murine pulp cell differentiation into odontoblast-like cells and stimulates biomineralization. J Endod 2012;38(9):1220–6.
70. Laurent P, Camps J, About I. Biodentine(TM) induces TGF-beta1 release from human pulp cells and early dental pulp mineralization. Int Endod J 2012;45(5): 439–48.

71. Tecles O, Laurent P, Aubut V, et al. Human tooth culture: a study model for reparative dentinogenesis and direct pulp capping materials biocompatibility. J Biomed Mater Res B Appl Biomater 2008;85(1):180–7.

72. Zhao X, He W, Song Z, et al. Mineral trioxide aggregate promotes odontoblastic differentiation via mitogen-activated protein kinase pathway in human dental pulp stem cells. Mol Biol Rep 2012;39(1):215–20.

73. Berger T, Baratz AZ, Gutmann JL. In vitro investigations into the etiology of mineral trioxide tooth staining. J Conserv Dent 2014;17(6):526–30.

74. Felman D, Parashos P. Coronal tooth discoloration and white mineral trioxide aggregate. J Endod 2013;39(4):484–7.

75. Krastl G, Allgayer N, Lenherr P, et al. Tooth discoloration induced by endodontic materials: a literature review. Dent Traumatol 2013;29(1):2–7.

76. Bortoluzzi EA, Araujo GS, Guerreiro Tanomaru JM, et al. Marginal gingiva discoloration by gray MTA: a case report. J Endod 2007;33(3):325–7.

77. Ioannidis K, Mistakidis I, Beltes P, et al. Spectrophotometric analysis of coronal discolouration induced by grey and white MTA. Int Endod J 2013;46(2):137–44.

78. Reynolds K, Johnson JD, Cohenca N. Pulp revascularization of necrotic bilateral bicuspids using a modified novel technique to eliminate potential coronal discolouration: a case report. Int Endod J 2009;42(1):84–92.

79. Keskin C, Demiryurek EO, Ozyurek T. Color stabilities of calcium silicate-based materials in contact with different irrigation solutions. J Endod 2015;41(3):409–11.

80. Camilleri J. Staining potential of neo MTA Plus, MTA Plus, and biodentine used for pulpotomy procedures. J Endod 2015;41(7):1139–45.

81. Valles M, Mercade M, Duran-Sindreu F, et al. Influence of light and oxygen on the color stability of five calcium silicate-based materials. J Endod 2013;39(4):525–8.

82. Valles M, Roig M, Duran-Sindreu F, et al. Color stability of teeth restored with biodentine: A 6-month in vitro study. J Endod 2015;41(7):1157–60.

83. Chen I, Salhab I, Setzer FC, et al. A new calcium silicate-based bioceramic material promotes human osteo- and odontogenic stem cell proliferation and survival via the extracellular signal-regulated kinase signaling pathway. J Endod 2016; 42(3):480–6.

84. Frank AL. Therapy for the divergent pulpless tooth by continued apical formation. J Am Dent Assoc 1966;72(1):87–93.

85. Diogenes A, Ruparel NB, Shiloah Y, et al. Regenerative endodontics: a way forward. J Am Dent Assoc 2016;147(5):372–80.

86. Alobaid AS, Cortes LM, Lo J, et al. Radiographic and clinical outcomes of the treatment of immature permanent teeth by revascularization or apexification: a pilot retrospective cohort study. J Endod 2014;40(8):1063–70.

87. Andreasen JO, Farik B, Munksgaard EC. Long-term calcium hydroxide as a root canal dressing may increase risk of root fracture. Dent Traumatol 2002;18(3): 134–7.

88. Fried K, Lillesaar C, Sime W, et al. Target finding of pain nerve fibers: neural growth mechanisms in the tooth pulp. Physiol Behav 2007;92(1–2):40–5.

89. Fried K, Nosrat C, Lillesaar C, et al. Molecular signaling and pulpal nerve development. Crit Rev Oral Biol Med 2000;11(3):318–32.

90. Huang GT, Sonoyama W, Liu Y, et al. The hidden treasure in apical papilla: the potential role in pulp/dentin regeneration and bioroot engineering. J Endod 2008;34(6):645–51.

91. de Almeida JF, Chen P, Henry MA, et al. Stem cells of the apical papilla regulate trigeminal neurite outgrowth and targeting through a BDNF-dependent mechanism. Tissue Eng Part A 2014;20(23–24):3089–100.

92. Iohara K, Imabayashi K, Ishizaka R, et al. Complete pulp regeneration after pulpectomy by transplantation of CD105+ stem cells with stromal cell-derived factor-1. Tissue Eng Part A 2011;17(15–16):1911–20.

93. Ishizaka R, Hayashi Y, Iohara K, et al. Stimulation of angiogenesis, neurogenesis and regeneration by side population cells from dental pulp. Biomaterials 2013; 34(8):1888–97.

94. Becerra P, Ricucci D, Loghin S, et al. Histologic study of a human immature permanent premolar with chronic apical abscess after revascularization/revitalization. J Endod 2014;40(1):133–9.

95. Shimizu E, Ricucci D, Albert J, et al. Clinical, radiographic, and histological observation of a human immature permanent tooth with chronic apical abscess after revitalization treatment. J Endod 2013;39(8):1078–83.

96. Martin G, Ricucci D, Gibbs JL, et al. Histological findings of revascularized/revitalized immature permanent molar with apical periodontitis using platelet-rich plasma. J Endod 2013;39(1):138–44.

97. Simon SR, Tomson PL, Berdal A. Regenerative endodontics: regeneration or repair? J Endod 2014;40(4 Suppl):S70–5.

98. Ishizaka R, Iohara K, Murakami M, et al. Regeneration of dental pulp following pulpectomy by fractionated stem/progenitor cells from bone marrow and adipose tissue. Biomaterials 2012;33(7):2109–18.

# Biological Molecules for the Regeneration of the Pulp-Dentin Complex

Sahng G. Kim, DDS, MS

## KEYWORDS

- Biological molecules • Signaling molecules • Growth factors • Biological cues
- Pulp-dentin complex • Tubular dentin • Odontoblast

## KEY POINTS

- The pulp-dentin complex plays a crucial role in fueling immune defense and tissue regeneration on infection or trauma.
- The regeneration of the pulp-dentin complex has been reported in several animal studies using exogenous biological cues or stem/progenitor cells.
- The animal and human studies using endogenous biological molecules released from ethylenediaminetetraacetic acid–conditioned dentin or evoked bleeding have shown the formation of tissues that are of periodontal origin.
- Endogenous biological molecules have a release profile with a high initial burst followed by rapid reduction, perhaps accounting for the lack of regeneration in clinical studies using current regenerative endodontic protocols.
- Delivery methods that allow for the controlled release of biological molecules may enhance the histologic outcome of regenerative endodontic therapy.

## INTRODUCTION

The pulp-dentin complex, as a dynamic functional structure in teeth, plays a pivotal role in the immune defense against noxious stimuli and tissue repair and regeneration during trauma and infection.[1] From a tissue engineering perspective, it is considered one of the most difficult tissues to regenerate because of its unique anatomic and physiologic nature. Unlike bone, which requires constant remodeling to maintain homeostasis, dentin rarely remodels in normal physiologic conditions. Only in pathologic conditions is dentin remodeling, such as resorption or repair, observed.[2] Dental pulp is a loose fibrous connective tissue but anatomically distinct from periodontal ligaments or other connective tissues in that it has functional odontoblasts to be coupled with dentin.

Disclosure Statement: The author has nothing to disclose. The author has no conflicts of interest related to this study.
Division of Endodontics, College of Dental Medicine, Columbia University, 630 West 168 Street, PH7Stem128, New York, NY 10032, USA
E-mail address: sgk2114@columbia.edu

Dent Clin N Am 61 (2017) 127–141
http://dx.doi.org/10.1016/j.cden.2016.08.005
0011-8532/17/© 2016 Elsevier Inc. All rights reserved.

A tenet of regenerative endodontic therapy is that dentin and pulp are anatomically restored to function as a physiologic unit, that is, the pulp-dentin complex. However, clinical regenerative endodontic treatment is not effective yet in the regeneration of the pulp-dentin complex.[3,4] The histologic observations in a few case reports showed that the regenerated tissues in infected necrotic teeth comprise mineralized tissues with the characteristics of bone and cementum and periodontal ligamentlike connective tissue.[3,4] In contrast, several animal studies found the robust pulp and dentin regeneration in pulp regeneration models using stem cells or biological molecules.[5-10]

The biological molecules, whether their source is endogenous or exogenous, control the cellular activities such as migration, proliferation, and differentiation so that homeostatic and regenerative needs in a specific tissue can be met during injury or infection. In regenerative endodontic therapy, endogenous signals can be released from conditioned dentin or bleeding evoked into the root canal. A few exogenous biological molecules to be most effective in pulp regeneration can be selected and introduced into the root canal in anticipation of energizing certain cellular behaviors toward robust pulp and dentin regeneration. The knowledge of how biological cues modulate cellular events during the pulp regeneration process is instrumental in identifying the limitations of clinical regenerative treatment and devising improved regeneration protocols. This review discusses the biological and clinical significance of regenerating the pulp-dentin complex, the role of biological molecules in pulp regeneration, the delivery limitation of biological molecules in current regenerative endodontic treatment, and the delivery methods of signaling molecules to direct cellular behaviors toward regeneration.

## THE SIGNIFICANCE OF REGENERATING THE PULP-DENTIN COMPLEX

The regenerated tissues in root canals after the application of clinical regeneration protocols seem to be of periodontal origin as evinced by the presence of periodontal ligamentlike, cementumlike, bonelike tissues in animal and human studies.[3,4,11-19] Notably, however, various clinical protocols used in regenerative endodontic treatment reliably have yielded the excellent clinical results such as healing of apical periodontitis, increased root lengths and thicknesses, or return of vitality.[20] The evidence inferred from histologic and clinical outcomes suggests that the radiographic findings from successful regenerative endodontic cases only reflect ectopic tissue formation in the root canal space.[3,4,11-19] From a clinical perspective, the need for regenerating the pulp-dentin complex may not be well justified if the goal of regenerative endodontic therapy is to prevent and cure apical periodontitis and to render immature necrotic teeth less susceptible to fracture by increasing the root volume. By contrast, from a biological standpoint, the pulp-dentin complex is crucial in activating the immune defense mechanisms and inducing the regeneration/repair on tissue injury or infection (**Fig. 1**). For instance, neuropeptides, such as substance P and calcitonin gene-related peptides, released from activated sensory nerves initiate neurogenic inflammation, availing the regeneration of the pulp-dentin complex by control of the immune responses and by stimulating tissue-forming cells.[21] Historically, the formation of fibrous connective tissue in the root canal space has been well documented since the earlier efforts by Ostby[22] and Nygaard-Ostby and Hjortdal,[23] but tubular dentin and odontoblastic layers to be regenerated in the context of immune defense and homeostasis have received less attention by researchers.

### Tubular Dentin

The tubular structure of dentin results from odontoblastic differentiation of the outer cells of dental papilla and subsequent dentin matrix deposition and its mineralization

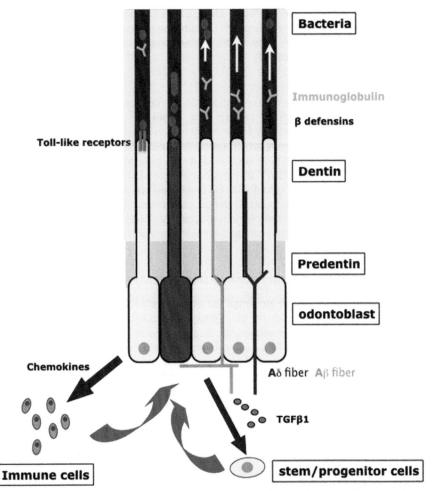

**Fig. 1.** The biological significance of the pulp-dentin complex at the time of injury or infection. The outward flow of dentinal fluid prevents the inward diffusion of bacteria on the exposure of dentinal tubules (*white arrows*). Immunoglobulins in dentinal fluid neutralize and opsonize bacteria. Beta-defensin released by odontoblasts kills bacteria and recruits other immune cells such as dendritic cells or lymphocytes. Sensory nerve fibers in dentinal tubules (Aβ and Aδ fibers) serve as an early warning system to safeguard the pulp from injuries. Toll-like receptors expressed on the membrane of odontoblasts recognize the specific pathogens and trigger the innate immunity. Odontoblasts release TGF β1, which triggers regeneration by modulating inflammation and recruiting stem/progenitor cells to the injury site.

during the tooth development. The dentinal tubules contain not only odontoblast processes but also dentinal fluid and sensory nerve fibers, which play a critical role in mounting the first line of defense along with odontoblasts underlying the tubular dentin. The outward flow of dentinal fluid prevents the inward diffusion of foreign substances such as bacteria and bacteria byproducts on the exposure of dentinal tubules.[24,25] Furthermore, immunoglobulins in dentinal fluid also function as deterrents of bacterial invasion.[26–28] Sensory nerve endings in dentinal tubules provide early detection of temperature change and mechanical stimuli and nociception to shield the pulp from injuries.[29,30] Despite the structural and biological significance of tubular dentin, its regeneration after regenerative endodontic treatment has not yet been shown (**Table 1**).

### Odontoblastic Layers

The regeneration of odontoblasts underlying dentin has been reported in a few animal studies using orthotopic animal models (see **Table 1**).[7–10] Odontoblasts not only secrete dentin matrix but also play a significant role as an immune cell.[31] Odontoblasts also express toll-like receptors, which recognize specific pathogens and trigger the recruitment of other immune cells such as dendritic cells and lymphocytes.[31,32] Other molecules including β-defensin[33] or transforming growth factor-β (TGF-β)[34] are also known to be released by odontoblasts. Beta-defensin seems to be bactericidal against bacteria commonly found in dental caries such as *Streptococcus mutans* and *Lactobacillus*.[33] TGF-β controls homeostasis by exerting proinflammatory effects during the early phase of injuries and anti-inflammatory and tissue-forming effects during the late stage.[34,35]

## BIOLOGICAL CUES FOR DENTAL PULP AND DENTIN REGENERATION

Tissue engineering strategies for dental pulp-dentin regeneration in preclinical animal studies include transplantation of stem/progenitor cells or use of biological molecules.[36] Clinical regenerative endodontic treatment uses the endogenous stem/progenitor cells from periapical tissues and biological molecules released from dentin[37] or evoked bleeding. The sources of biological cues include endogenous growth factors from conditioned dentin or apical bleeding and exogenous signaling molecules. In addition, stem/progenitor cells transplanted into the root canals or migrated from periapical tissues during evoked bleeding participate in the regeneration processes

**Table 1**
**Histologic findings after regenerative endodontic therapy in animal and human studies**

| Study | Type of Study | Tubular Dentin | Odontoblastic Layers | Ectopic Tissues |
|---|---|---|---|---|
| Thibodeau et al,[11] 2007 | Animal | No | No | Yes |
| Wang et al,[12] 2010 | Animal | No | No | Yes |
| Iohara et al,[7] 2011 | Animal | No | Yes | No |
| Yamauchi et al,[13] 2011 | Animal | No | No | Yes |
| Ishizaka et al,[8] 2012 | Animal | No | Yes | No |
| Shimizu et al,[42] 2012 | Human | No | Yes | No |
| Zhu et al,[14] 2012 | Animal | No | No | Yes |
| Iohara et al,[9] 2013 | Animal | No | Yes | No |
| Tawfik et al,[15] 2013 | Animal | No | No | Yes |
| Gomes-Filho et al,[16] 2013 | Animal | No | No | Yes |
| Becerra et al,[3] 2014 | Human | No | No | Yes |
| Iohara et al,[10] 2014 | Animal | No | Yes | No |
| Torabinejad et al,[17] 2014 | Animal | No | No | Yes |
| Torabinejad et al,[18] 2015 | Animal | No | No | Yes |
| Saoud et al,[19] 2015 | Animal | No | No | Yes |
| Lei et al,[4] 2015 | Human | No | No | Yes |

not only by being incorporated in the differentiated tissues but also by releasing trophic factors,[38] which also function as biological signals.

### Preclinical Animal Studies

Animal studies using ectopic models have generally shown the regeneration of the pulp-dentin complex. In a study by Cordeiro and colleagues,[39] pulp-extirpated tooth slices were infused with stem cells from human exfoliated deciduous teeth (SHED) or human dermal microvascular endothelial cells in poly-L-lactic acid (PLLA) synthetic scaffold and implanted into the subcutaneous tissue of immunodeficient mice. The odontoblastic layers with tubular dentin were histologically observed in the tooth slices harvested 2 to 4 weeks after implantation.[39] The cell lineage tracing of transplanted SHED found that SHED differentiated into odontoblastlike cells and endothelial cells.[39] In a study by Huang and colleagues,[40] emptied root canals in tooth fragments were seeded with stem cells of the apical papilla and dental pulp stem cells (DPSC) in poly(D,L-lactide-co-glycolide) scaffolds and implanted into the subcutaneous tissue of severe combined immunodeficient mice. Histologic analysis of the tooth fragments extracted 3 to 4 months after implantation found the formation of odontoblastlike cells along the regenerated dentin with no evident tubular structures.[40] Galler and colleagues[5] also showed similar findings in an ectopic model using dentin cylinders. The dentin cylinders pretreated with ethylenediaminetetraacetic acid (EDTA) were filled with hydrogels containing vascular endothelial growth factors (VEGF), TGF-β1, and fibroblast growth factor-2 (FGF-2) as well as DPSC and then implanted into the dorsum of immunodeficient mice.[5] The retrieved implants 6 weeks after surgery showed the odontoblastlike cells and their processes extended into the dentinal tubules.[5] Ruangsawasdi and colleagues[41] found that odontoblastlike cell layers with strong immunoactivity of dentin sialoproteins were observed when premolars with emptied root canals were infused with fibrin gels and transplanted in the subcutaneous tissue above the rat calvaria. Horibe and colleagues[6] used the subpopulation of dental pulp stem cells (MDPSC) that were mobilized in response to granulocyte colony-stimulating factor (G-CSF) with a collagen scaffold to fill the pulpectomized human tooth roots and implanted the roots into the subcutaneous tissue of severe combined immunodeficient mice. Histologic data from harvested teeth 3 weeks after surgery showed tubular dentin lined with odontoblastlike cells.[6]

In orthotopic pulp regeneration models, the regeneration of dental pulp and dentin is not as commonly achieved as in ectopic models. Thibodeau and colleagues[11] showed ectopic mineralized tissue formation in the root canals 3 months after bleeding was evoked in a dog model with prior infection. Disinfection in this infection model included use of 1.25% sodium hypochlorite without mechanical instrumentation and triple antibiotic pastes.[11] The other group with the addition of collagen solution did not significantly enhance the histologic outcomes.[11] Wang and colleagues[12] also showed that the ectopic tissues composed of cementumlike and bonelike tissues scattered in the root canals or integrated into the native dentin and periodontal ligamentlike tissue were formed in the root canals in an infected dog model using a similar disinfection protocol. The ectopic tissue formation was identified in another dog study by Gomes-Filho and colleagues[16] using a similar disinfection protocol as shown in other studies with prior infection. Other factors including platelet-rich plasma (PRP) or bone marrow aspirate were also added after bleeding was induced but did not enhance the histologic outcome.[16] Saoud and colleagues[19] also showed the formation of periodontal ligamentlike, cementumlike, and bonelike tissues in a dog model with infected root canals. Similar histologic findings were presented by Tawfik and colleagues[15] in an infected dog model after disinfection using triple antibiotic paste and evoked bleeding with or without the addition of an FGF-2–loaded gelatin hydrogel scaffold. Torabinejad and colleagues[17,18] showed the ectopic tissue formation in a ferret model with previously infected root canals after PRP or blood clot/Gelfoam was used.

A series of studies by Nakashima and colleagues[7–10] using noninfected dog models found the regeneration of dentin and odontoblastic layers. Iohara and colleagues[7] transplanted the subpopulation of stem/progenitor cells (CD105[+]) isolated from pulp and adipose tissue in pulpectomized dog incisors with complete apical closure. The apical foramen was enlarged to 0.7 mm in diameter before the transplantation of CD105[+] cells and collagen scaffold with or without stromal-derived factor-1 (SDF-1).[7] The transplantation of pulp CD105[+] cells with SDF-1 yielded the regeneration of almost complete pulp tissue in 90 days after surgery, which was significantly greater than that of other groups including adipose CD105[+] cells with SDF-1 and CD105[+] cells only.[7] Odontoblastlike layers were observed, although the tubular structure of dentin was not clearly identified.[7] Ishizaka and colleagues[8] used CD31[−] side population (SP) cells isolated from dental pulp, bone marrow, and adipose tissue in dog teeth prepared in the same manner. The transplantation of pulp CD31[−] SP cells with SDF-1 yielded approximately 45% of pulp tissue regeneration 28 days after surgery, which was significantly greater than that of bone marrow CD31[−] SP cells but not significantly different from that of adipose CD31[−] SP cells.[8] Iohara and colleagues[9,10] transplanted MDPSC and G-CSF–laden collagen scaffold into the emptied root canals in dog incisors with an apical foramen enlarged to 0.5 mm[10] or 0.6 mm[9] in diameter and yielded more than 90% pulp tissue regeneration 60 days after surgery in young (8–10 months old) dogs and approximately 60% pulp tissue regeneration 120 days after surgery in aged (5–6 years old) dogs.

### Clinical Studies

Histologic assessment was performed in a few case reports in which a tooth was extracted for an orthodontic reason or because of a tooth fracture.[3,4,42] The clinical cases showed that tissues formed in the root canals were of periodontal origin as histologically visualized in several orthotopic animal studies with artificially induced apical periodontitis.[3,4] Only one clinical case with irreversible pulpitis reported distinct odontoblastic layers along the native dentin without ectopic tissue formation after regenerative endodontic treatment.[42] Bleeding was induced in all clinical studies showing histologic findings,[3,4,42] but only Lei and colleagues[4] used 17% EDTA before evoked bleeding.

### Endogenous Biological Cues

Dentin contains a variety of biological molecules including growth factors,[37,43–45] noncollagenous proteins,[46] and glycosaminoglycans.[47,48] The growth factors such as TGF-β1,[44,45] bone morphogenetic protein (BMP),[49,50] growth/differentiation factor (GDF),[51] FGF-2,[52] VEGF,[52] insulinlike growth factor (IGF),[43,51] and platelet-derived growth factor (PDGF)[44] can be released from dentin at the time of dentin demineralization. Noncollagenous proteins in dentin include dentin sialoprotein,[53] dentin phosphoprotein,[54,55] dentin matrix protein,[56–58] bone sialoprotein,[59] and osteopontin.[60,61] Sulfated glycosaminoglycans[47,48] such as chondroitin sulfates and dermatan sulfates are also found in dentin matrix.

The dentin matrix molecules are liberated when demineralization occurs.[45] During the regenerative endodontic procedure, EDTA is used to demineralize dentin as a chelating agent before the influx of endogenous stem/progenitor cells so that the biological cues embedded in dentin matrix can be released and direct the cellular activities toward regeneration. The biological effects of these molecules[62–91] are summarized in **Table 2**. Presumably, apical bleeding delivers the biological molecules to the root canal space along with stem/progenitor cells[92] because blood clots contain blood-derived growth factors such as PDGF, TGF-β, FGF, VEGF, and IGF. The endogenous factors are thought to fuel the activities of recruited cells and pulp regeneration.

## Exogenous Biological Cues

All individual growth factors that exist in dentin matrix and apical bleeding can be potential candidates for biological cues to be exogenously transplanted. The exogenous biological molecules are not different from the endogenous counterparts in their biological effects. However, a few select exogenous biological factors with higher concentrations may augment the regeneration processes. For example, PRP is known to have higher concentrations of blood-derived factors compared with those of apical bleeding[93] and has been used in the hope of enhancing the clinical and histologic outcome.[14,16–18]

The signaling molecules to be considered as exogenous biological cues for pulp regeneration should precisely control cell migration, cell proliferation, odontoblastic differentiation, angiogenesis, and neurogenesis. The signaling molecules that play a role in cell migration are TGF-β1,[62] FGF-2,[79] SDF-1,[94,95] and PDGF.[44] Cell proliferation is promoted by TGF-β1,[63] FGF-2,[64] PDGF,[88,89] and IGF.[86] Odontoblastic differentiation and dentinogenesis are induced by TGF-β1,[64,65] PDGF,[90] BMP-2,[66–71] BMP-4,[69–71] BMP-7,[72–76] GDF,[77,78] FGF-2,[80–82] IGF,[86] and nerve growth factor.[96] Angiogenesis is

| Table 2 | |
| :--- | :--- |
| **Biological effects of dentin matrix molecules** | |
| **Dentin Matrix Molecules** | **Biological Effects** |
| Growth factors | |
| TGF-β1[44,45] | Chemotaxis,[62] cell proliferation,[63] odontoblastic differentiation,[64] dentinogenesis[65] |
| BMP-2[49] | Odontoblastic differentiation,[66–70] dentinogenesis[69–71] |
| BMP-4[49] | Odontoblastic differentiation,[70] dentinogenesis[69–71] |
| BMP-7[50] | Dentinogenesis[72–76] |
| GDF[51] | Odontoblastic differentiation,[77,78] dentinogenesis[77,78] |
| FGF-2[52] | Chemotaxis,[79] cell proliferation,[64] dentinogenesis[80–82] |
| VEGF[52] | Cell proliferation,[83] angiogenesis[84,85] |
| IGF[43,51] | Cell proliferation,[86] odontoblastic differentiation[86] |
| PDGF[44] | Cell migration,[87] cell proliferation,[88,89] dentin matrix synthesis,[88,89] odontoblastic differentiation,[90] angiogenesis[91] |
| Noncollagenous proteins | |
| DSP[53] | Not determined |
| DPP[54,55] | Dentinogenesis[54,55] |
| DMP[56–58] | Dentinogenesis[56–58] |
| BSP[59] | Dentinogenesis[59] |
| OPN[60,61] | Inhibition of dentinogenesis[60,61] |
| Glycosaminoglycans | |
| Chondroitin sulfate[47,48] | Dentinogenesis[47,48] |
| Dermatan sulfate[47,48] | Dentinogenesis[47,48] |

*Abbreviations:* BSP, bone sialoprotein; DMP, dentin matrix protein; DPP, dentin phosphoprotein; DSP, dentin sialoprotein; OPN, osteopontin.

stimulated by VEGF,[84,85] and PDGF.[91] The growth, survival and maintenance of neurons are regulated by nerve growth factor.[97,98] Several animal studies delivered these growth factors with stem/progenitor cells to control the behaviors of the transplanted cells. For example, SDF-1 was transplanted with CD105$^+$ or CD31$^-$ SP cells in the root canals of dog incisors.[7,8] SDF-1, a strong chemotactic agent, was strategically placed in the coronal root canals on top of the transplanted cells to further the migration of the transplantation.[7,8] G-CSF, which is potent in recruiting MDPSCs, was used for the same reason in other orthotopic animal models.[9,10]

## DELIVERY OF BIOLOGICAL MOLECULES

### Release Profile of Biological Molecules and Its Implications for Pulp Regeneration

The release profiles and biological effects of growth factors play a crucial role for controlling the cell behaviors that are required at the different stages of pulp regeneration. The release profile of a growth factor can dictate its biological effect. Kikuchi and colleagues[82] found that a favorable healing pattern was observed when FGF-2 was released in a controlled manner as evidenced by the direction of dentin formation. Controlled release can be referred to as the release of a biological factor at a specific rate within a certain period. If a biological molecule is delivered or released without the help of a carrier or a scaffold that allows for controlled release, its biological effect is abated in a short period. At the early stage of regeneration, cell mobilization is predominant, whereas at the later stage, cell differentiation and tissue formation are. Therefore, the biological molecules involved in cell differentiation and tissue formation should have a controlled release profile so that the biological effects can be sustained during the later stage of regeneration. In contrast, the controlled release of cell migratory factors may not be as critical, as their effects are limited to the initial phase of regeneration.

### Delivery Limitation of Biological Cues in Current Regenerative Endodontic Treatment

Endogenous biological molecules from EDTA-conditioned dentin[45] or blood clots[93] in current regenerative endodontic treatment suffer from uncontrolled release. Namely, biological factors released from dentin or evoked bleeding has a release profile with a high initial burst followed by rapid reduction. Therefore, they may not be available at the later stage of pulp regeneration, when critical biological events such as differentiation and tissue formation are to be coordinated. The unavailability of biological molecules at the critical tissue-forming stages may account for the ectopic tissue formation in the root canal space in human and animal studies.[3,4,11–19] Furthermore, as discussed above, the amount and concentrations of endogenous biological cues are not as high as those of exogenous growth factors and may not be sufficient to control or augment a certain cellular activity during tissue regeneration.

### Delivery Methods of Biological Molecules

For biological molecules to be functional throughout the regenerative processes, biological molecules need to be incorporated into biodegradable scaffolds. This process is called *scaffold functionalization*. Because the biological molecules are released while the scaffolds degrade, the degradation time of a scaffold is crucial for their biological effects, and it is suggested to be at least 2 months based on the regeneration rates of pulp tissues in orthotopic animal studies.[7–10] Collagen matrix commonly used in current regenerative endodontic therapy has a degradation time of approximately 2 weeks and cannot deliver the biological cues during the late stage of pulp regeneration.

Microspheres containing growth factors are another suitable delivery vehicle of growth factors, as the growth factors can be released in a controlled manner similar to that of the functionalized scaffolds. The more sophisticated delivery method of growth factors is core/shell microspheres.[99–101] In core/shell microspheres, 2 different growth factors are separately encapsulated in the 2 compartments of the microspheres: core (inner compartment) and shell (outer compartment). During the erosion of the microspheres, the growth factor in the outer compartment is released first, and then the growth factor in the inner compartment can be released. This sequential release of 2 growth factors in the core/shell microspheres is beneficial to exert a strategic control of cellular events. For instance, the growth factors that are essential at the later stages of pulp regeneration are encapsulated in the core, whereas the factors that are useful at the early stage of pulp regeneration are incorporated in the shell. The core/shell microspheres can be designed to have different combinations of growth factors so that the regeneration processes may be precisely controlled by the release of specific biological cues at different time points.

## SUMMARY

The regeneration of the pulp-dentin complex has significant biological implications in the context of the immune defense and homeostasis. The current regenerative endodontic therapy has not yielded the regeneration of dental pulp and dentin characterized by the presence of tubular dentin and odontoblastic layers. The regeneration of the pulp-dentin complex has been commonly reported in ectopic animal models and has been rarely demonstrated in orthotopic animal models. A careful assessment of dissimilar histologic outcomes among orthotopic animal models has found that use of current regeneration protocols is not conducive to the regeneration of the pulp-dentin complex, perhaps because of the ineffective delivery method of biological molecules or inefficient disinfection protocols. On the other hand, several animal studies using cell transplantation and exogenous biological molecules have demonstrated the pulplike and dentinlike tissues with functional odontoblastic layers. For a biological cue to be functional during pulp tissue regeneration, the delivery of biological molecules requires a scaffold or a carrier that allows for controlled release. Endogenous biological molecules seem to be released from dentin matrix or apical bleeding in an uncontrolled manner during the regenerative processes. The functionalized biodegradable scaffolds or microspheres that allow the controlled release of growth factors may be useful in regenerative endodontic treatment to divert the cellular events toward regeneration rather than repair.

## REFERENCES

1. Pashley DH. Dynamics of the pulpo-dentin complex. Crit Rev Oral Biol Med 1996;7(2):104–33.
2. Zheng Y, Chen M, He L, et al. Mesenchymal dental pulp cells attenuate dentin resorption in homeostasis. J Dent Res 2015;94(6):821–7.
3. Becerra P, Ricucci D, Loghin S, et al. Histologic study of a human immature permanent premolar with chronic apical abscess after revascularization/revitalization. J Endod 2014;40(1):133–9.
4. Lei L, Chen Y, Zhou R, et al. Histologic and immunohistochemical findings of a human immature permanent tooth with apical periodontitis after regenerative endodontic treatment. J Endod 2015;41(7):1172–9.
5. Galler KM, D'Souza RN, Federlin M, et al. Dentin conditioning codetermines cell fate in regenerative endodontics. J Endod 2011;37(11):1536–41.

6. Horibe H, Murakami M, Iohara K, et al. Isolation of a stable subpopulation of mobilized dental pulp stem cells (MDPSCs) with high proliferation, migration, and regeneration potential is independent of age. PLoS One 2014;9(5):e98553.

7. Iohara K, Imabayashi K, Ishizaka R, et al. Complete pulp regeneration after pulpectomy by transplantation of CD105+ stem cells with stromal cell-derived factor-1. Tissue Eng Part A 2011;17(15–16):1911–20.

8. Ishizaka R, Iohara K, Murakami M, et al. Regeneration of dental pulp following pulpectomy by fractionated stem/progenitor cells from bone marrow and adipose tissue. Biomaterials 2012;33(7):2109–18.

9. Iohara K, Murakami M, Takeuchi N, et al. A novel combinatorial therapy with pulp stem cells and granulocyte colony-stimulating factor for total pulp regeneration. Stem Cells Transl Med 2013;2(7):521–33.

10. Iohara K, Murakami M, Nakata K, et al. Age-dependent decline in dental pulp regeneration after pulpectomy in dogs. Exp Gerontol 2014;52:39–45.

11. Thibodeau B, Teixeira F, Yamauchi M, et al. Pulp revascularization of immature dog teeth with apical periodontitis. J Endod 2007;33(6):680–9.

12. Wang X, Thibodeau B, Trope M, et al. Histologic characterization of regenerated tissues in canal space after the revitalization/revascularization procedure of immature dog teeth with apical periodontitis. J Endod 2010;36(1):56–63.

13. Yamauchi N, Nagaoka H, Yamauchi S, et al. Immunohistological characterization of newly formed tissues after regenerative procedure in immature dog teeth. J Endod 2011;37(12):1636–41.

14. Zhu X, Zhang C, Huang GT, et al. Transplantation of dental pulp stem cells and platelet-rich plasma for pulp regeneration. J Endod 2012;38(12):1604–9.

15. Tawfik H, Abu-Seida AM, Hashem AA, et al. Regenerative potential following revascularization of immature permanent teeth with necrotic pulps. Int Endod J 2013;46(10):910–22.

16. Gomes-Filho JE, Duarte PC, Ervolino E, et al. Histologic characterization of engineered tissues in the canal space of closed-apex teeth with apical periodontitis. J Endod 2013;39(12):1549–56.

17. Torabinejad M, Faras H, Corr R, et al. Histologic examinations of teeth treated with 2 scaffolds: a pilot animal investigation. J Endod 2014;40(4):515–20.

18. Torabinejad M, Milan M, Shabahang S, et al. Histologic examination of teeth with necrotic pulps and periapical lesions treated with 2 scaffolds: an animal investigation. J Endod 2015;41(6):846–52.

19. Saoud TM, Zaazou A, Nabil A, et al. Histological observations of pulpal replacement tissue in immature dog teeth after revascularization of infected pulps. Dent Traumatol 2015;31(3):243–9.

20. Kontakiotis EG, Filippatos CG, Tzanetakis GN, et al. Regenerative endodontic therapy: a data analysis of clinical protocols. J Endod 2015;41(2):146–54.

21. Caviedes-Bucheli J, Muñoz HR, Azuero-Holguín MM, et al. Neuropeptides in dental pulp: the silent protagonists. J Endod 2008;34(7):773–88.

22. OSTBY BN. The role of the blood clot in endodontic therapy. An experimental histologic study. Acta Odontol Scand 1961;19:324–53.

23. Nygaard-Ostby B, Hjortdal O. Tissue formation in the root canal following pulp removal. Scand J Dent Res 1971;79(5):333–49.

24. Maita E, Simpson MD, Tao L, et al. Fluid and protein flux across the pulpodentine complex of the dog in vivo. Arch Oral Biol 1991;36(2):103–10.

25. Pashley DH. The influence of dentin permeability and pulpal blood flow on pulpal solute concentrations. J Endod 1979;5(12):355–61.

26. Pulver WH, Taubman MA, Smith DJ. Immune components in normal and in-flamed human dental pulp. Arch Oral Biol 1977;22(2):103–11.
27. Okamura K. Histological study on the origin of dentinal immunoglobulins and the change in their localization during caries. J Oral Pathol 1985;14(9):680–9.
28. Hahn CL, Best AM. The pulpal origin of immunoglobulins in dentin beneath caries: an immunohistochemical study. J Endod 2006;32(3):178–82.
29. Byers MR. Dental sensory receptors. Int Rev Neurobiol 1984;25:39–94.
30. Byers MR, Närhi MV. Dental injury models: experimental tools for understanding neuroinflammatory interactions and polymodal nociceptor functions. Crit Rev Oral Biol Med 1999;10(1):4–39.
31. Couve E, Osorio R, Schmachtenberg O. The amazing odontoblast: activity, autophagy, and aging. J Dent Res 2013;92(9):765–72.
32. Durand SH, Flacher V, Roméas A, et al. Lipoteichoic acid increases TLR and functional chemokine expression while reducing dentin formation in in vitro differentiated human odontoblasts. J Immunol 2006;176(5):2880–7.
33. Shiba H, Mouri Y, Komatsuzawa H, et al. Macrophage inflammatory protein-3alpha and beta-defensin-2 stimulate dentin sialophosphoprotein gene expression in human pulp cells. Biochem Biophys Res Commun 2003;306(4):867–71.
34. Sloan AJ, Perry H, Matthews JB, et al. Transforming growth factor-beta isoform expression in mature human healthy and carious molar teeth. Histochem J 2000;32(4):247–52.
35. Piattelli A, Rubini C, Fioroni M, et al. Transforming growth factor-beta 1 (TGF-beta 1) expression in normal healthy pulps and in those with irreversible pulpitis. Int Endod J 2004;37(2):114–9.
36. Kim SG, Zheng Y, Zhou J, et al. Dentin and dental pulp regeneration by the patient's endogenous cells. Endod Topics 2013;28(1):106–17.
37. Smith AJ, Duncan HF, Diogenes A, et al. Exploiting the bioactive properties of the dentin-pulp complex in regenerative endodontics. J Endod 2016;42(1):47–56.
38. Yamamoto T, Osako Y, Ito M, et al. Trophic effects of dental pulp stem cells on schwann cells in peripheral nerve regeneration. Cell Transplant 2016;25(1):183–93.
39. Cordeiro MM, Dong Z, Kaneko T, et al. Dental pulp tissue engineering with stem cells from exfoliated deciduous teeth. J Endod 2008;34(8):962–9.
40. Huang GT, Yamaza T, Shea LD, et al. Stem/progenitor cell-mediated de novo regeneration of dental pulp with newly deposited continuous layer of dentin in an in vivo model. Tissue Eng Part A 2010;16(2):605–15.
41. Ruangsawasdi N, Zehnder M, Weber FE. Fibrin gel improves tissue ingrowth and cell differentiation in human immature premolars implanted in rats. J Endod 2014;40(2):246–50.
42. Shimizu E, Jong G, Partridge N, et al. Histologic observation of a human immature permanent tooth with irreversible pulpitis after revascularization/regeneration procedure. J Endod 2012;38(9):1293–7.
43. Finkelman RD, Mohan S, Jennings JC, et al. Quantitation of growth factors IGF-I, SGF/IGF-II, and TGF-beta in human dentin. J Bone Miner Res 1990;5(7):717–23.
44. Cassidy N, Fahey M, Prime SS, et al. Comparative analysis of transforming growth factor-beta isoforms 1-3 in human and rabbit dentine matrices. Arch Oral Biol 1997;42(3):219–23.
45. Galler KM, Buchalla W, Hiller KA, et al. Influence of root canal disinfectants on growth factor release from dentin. J Endod 2015;41(3):363–8.

46. Salehi S, Cooper P, Smith A, et al. Dentin matrix components extracted with phosphoric acid enhance cell proliferation and mineralization. Dent Mater 2016;32(3):334–42.

47. Nishikawa H, Ueno A, Nishikawa S, et al. Sulfated glycosaminoglycan synthesis and its regulation by transforming growth factor-beta in rat clonal dental pulp cells. J Endod 2000;26(3):169–71.

48. Garg HG, Joseph PA, Thompson BT, et al. Effect of fully sulfated glycosamino-glycans on pulmonary artery smooth muscle cell proliferation. Arch Biochem Biophys 1999;371(2):228–33.

49. Thomadakis G, Ramoshebi LN, Crooks J, et al. Immunolocalization of bone morphogenetic protein-2 and -3 and osteogenic Protein-1 during murine tooth root morphogenesis and in other craniofacial structures. Eur J Oral Sci 1999; 107(5):368–77.

50. Helder MN, Karg H, Bervoets TJ, et al. Bone morphogenetic protein-7 (osteo-genic protein-1, OP-1) and tooth development. J Dent Res 1998;77(4):545–54.

51. Duncan HF, Smith AJ, Fleming GJ, et al. Release of bio-active dentine extracel-lular matrix components by histone deacetylase inhibitors (HDACi). Int Endod J 2015 [Epub ahead of print]. Available at: http://www.ncbi.nlm.nih.gov/pubmed/26609946.

52. Roberts-Clark DJ, Smith AJ. Angiogenic growth factors in human dentine matrix. Arch Oral Biol 2000;45(11):1013–6.

53. Butler WT, Bhown M, Brunn JC, et al. Isolation, characterization and immunoloc-alization of a 53-kDal dentin sialoprotein (DSP). Matrix 1992;12(5):343–51.

54. Boskey AL, Maresca M, Doty S, et al. Concentration-dependent effects of dentin phosphophoryn in the regulation of in vitro hydroxyapatite formation and growth. Bone Miner 1990;11(1):55–65.

55. Saito T, Arsenault AL, Yamauchi M, et al. Mineral induction by immobilized phos-phoproteins. Bone 1997;21(4):305–11.

56. Tartaix PH, Doulaverakis M, George A, et al. In vitro effects of dentin matrix protein-1 on hydroxyapatite formation provide insights into in vivo functions. J Biol Chem 2004;279(18):18115–20.

57. He G, Gajjeraman S, Schultz D, et al. Spatially and temporally controlled biomin-eralization is facilitated by interaction between self-assembled dentin matrix protein 1 and calcium phosphate nuclei in solution. Biochemistry 2005;44(49): 16140–8.

58. Gajjeraman S, Narayanan K, Hao J, et al. Matrix macromolecules in hard tissues control the nucleation and hierarchical assembly of hydroxyapatite. J Biol Chem 2007;282(2):1193–204.

59. Hunter GK, Goldberg HA. Nucleation of hydroxyapatite by bone sialoprotein. Proc Natl Acad Sci U S A 1993;90(18):8562–5.

60. Boskey AL, Spevak L, Paschalis E, et al. Osteopontin deficiency increases min-eral content and mineral crystallinity in mouse bone. Calcif Tissue Int 2002; 71(2):145–54.

61. Hunter GK, Kyle CL, Goldberg HA. Modulation of crystal formation by bone phosphoproteins: structural specificity of the osteopontin-mediated inhibition of hydroxyapatite formation. Biochem J 1994;300(Pt 3):723–8.

62. Howard C, Murray PE, Namerow KN. Dental pulp stem cell migration. J Endod 2010;36(12):1963–6.

63. Melin M, Joffre-Romeas A, Farges JC, et al. Effects of TGFbeta1 on dental pulp cells in cultured human tooth slices. J Dent Res 2000;79(9):1689–96.

64. He H, Yu J, Liu Y, et al. Effects of FGF2 and TGFbeta1 on the differentiation of human dental pulp stem cellss in vitro. Cell Biol Int 2008;32(7):827–34.

65. Tziafas D, Papadimitriou S. Role of exogenous TGF-beta in induction of reparative dentinogenesis in vivo. Eur J Oral Sci 1998;106(Suppl 1):192–6.

66. Saito T, Ogawa M, Hata Y, et al. Acceleration effect of human recombinant bone morphogenetic protein-2 on differentiation of human pulp cells into odontoblasts. J Endod 2004;30(4):205–8.

67. Chen S, Gluhak-Heinrich J, Martinez M, et al. Bone morphogenetic protein 2 mediates dentin sialophosphoprotein expression and odontoblast differentiation via NF-Y signaling. J Biol Chem 2008;283(28):19359–70.

68. Iohara K, Nakashima M, Ito M, et al. Dentin regeneration by dental pulp stem cell therapy with recombinant human bone morphogenetic protein 2. J Dent Res 2004;83(8):590–5.

69. Nakashima M. Induction of dentin formation on canine amputated pulp by recombinant human bone morphogenetic proteins (BMP)-2 and -4. J Dent Res 1994;73(9):1515–22.

70. Nakashima M, Nagasawa H, Yamada Y, et al. Regulatory role of transforming growth factor-beta, bone morphogenetic protein-2, and protein-4 on gene expression of extracellular matrix proteins and differentiation of dental pulp cells. Dev Biol 1994;162(1):18–28.

71. Nakashima M. Induction of dentine in amputated pulp of dogs by recombinant human bone morphogenetic proteins-2 and -4 with collagen matrix. Arch Oral Biol 1994;39(12):1085–9.

72. Rutherford RB, Gu K. Treatment of inflamed ferret dental pulps with recombinant bone morphogenetic protein-7. Eur J Oral Sci 2000;108(3):202–6.

73. Rutherford RB, Spångberg L, Tucker M, et al. The time-course of the induction of reparative dentine formation in monkeys by recombinant human osteogenic protein-1. Arch Oral Biol 1994;39(10):833–8.

74. Rutherford RB, Wahle J, Tucker M, et al. Induction of reparative dentine formation in monkeys by recombinant human osteogenic protein-1. Arch Oral Biol 1993;38(7):571–6.

75. Six N, Lasfargues JJ, Goldberg M. Differential repair responses in the coronal and radicular areas of the exposed rat molar pulp induced by recombinant human bone morphogenetic protein 7 (osteogenic protein 1). Arch Oral Biol 2002; 47(3):177–87.

76. Jepsen S, Albers HK, Fleiner B, et al. Recombinant human osteogenic protein-1 induces dentin formation: an experimental study in miniature swine. J Endod 1997;23(6):378–82.

77. Nakashima M, Iohara K, Ishikawa M, et al. Stimulation of reparative dentin formation by ex vivo gene therapy using dental pulp stem cells electrotransfected with growth/differentiation factor 11 (Gdf11). Hum Gene Ther 2004;15(11): 1045–53.

78. Nakashima M, Tachibana K, Iohara K, et al. Induction of reparative dentin formation by ultrasound-mediated gene delivery of growth/differentiation factor 11. Hum Gene Ther 2003;14(6):591–7.

79. Suzuki T, Lee CH, Chen M, et al. Induced migration of dental pulp stem cells for in vivo pulp regeneration. J Dent Res 2011;90(8):1013–8.

80. Kitamura C, Nishihara T, Terashita M, et al. Local regeneration of dentin-pulp complex using controlled release of fgf-2 and naturally derived sponge-like scaffolds. Int J Dent 2012;2012:190561.

81. Ishimatsu H, Kitamura C, Morotomi T, et al. Formation of dentinal bridge on surface of regenerated dental pulp in dentin defects by controlled release of fibroblast growth factor-2 from gelatin hydrogels. J Endod 2009;35(6):858–65.

82. Kikuchi N, Kitamura C, Morotomi T, et al. Formation of dentin-like particles in dentin defects above exposed pulp by controlled release of fibroblast growth factor 2 from gelatin hydrogels. J Endod 2007;33(10):1198–202.

83. D'Alimonte I, Nargi E, Mastrangelo F, et al. Vascular endothelial growth factor enhances in vitro proliferation and osteogenic differentiation of human dental pulp stem cells. J Biol Regul Homeost Agents 2011;25(1):57–69.

84. Leung DW, Cachianes G, Kuang WJ, et al. Vascular endothelial growth factor is a secreted angiogenic mitogen. Science 1989;246(4935):1306–9.

85. Zhang Z, Nor F, Oh M, et al. Wnt/βcatenin signaling determines the vasculogenic fate of post-natal mesenchymal stem cells. Stem Cells 2016;34(6):1576–87.

86. Onishi T, Kinoshita S, Shintani S, et al. Stimulation of proliferation and differentiation of dog dental pulp cells in serum-free culture medium by insulin-like growth factor. Arch Oral Biol 1999;44(4):361–71.

87. Seppä H, Grotendorst G, Seppä S, et al. Platelet-derived growth factor in chemotactic for fibroblasts. J Cell Biol 1982;92(2):584–8.

88. Denholm IA, Moule AJ, Bartold PM. The behaviour and proliferation of human dental pulp cell strains in vitro, and their response to the application of platelet-derived growth factor-BB and insulin-like growth factor-1. Int Endod J 1998;31(4):251–8.

89. Nakashima M. The effects of growth factors on DNA synthesis, proteoglycan synthesis and alkaline phosphatase activity in bovine dental pulp cells. Arch Oral Biol 1992;37(3):231–6.

90. Yokose S, Kadokura H, Tajima N, et al. Platelet-derived growth factor exerts disparate effects on odontoblast differentiation depending on the dimers in rat dental pulp cells. Cell Tissue Res 2004;315(3):375–84.

91. Hellberg C, Ostman A, Heldin CH. PDGF and vessel maturation. Recent Results Cancer Res 2010;180:103–14.

92. Lovelace TW, Henry MA, Hargreaves KM, et al. Evaluation of the delivery of mesenchymal stem cells into the root canal space of necrotic immature teeth after clinical regenerative endodontic procedure. J Endod 2011;37(2):133–8.

93. Pietrzak WS, Eppley BL. Platelet rich plasma: biology and new technology. J Craniofac Surg 2005;16(6):1043–54.

94. Iohara K, Zheng L, Wake H, et al. A novel stem cell source for vasculogenesis in ischemia: subfraction of side population cells from dental pulp. Stem Cells 2008;26(9):2408–18.

95. Iohara K, Zheng L, Ito M, et al. Regeneration of dental pulp after pulpotomy by transplantation of CD31(-)/CD146(-) side population cells from a canine tooth. Regen Med 2009;4(3):377–85.

96. Arany S, Koyota S, Sugiyama T. Nerve growth factor promotes differentiation of odontoblast-like cells. J Cell Biochem 2009;106(4):539–45.

97. Woodnutt DA, Wager-Miller J, O'Neill PC, et al. Neurotrophin receptors and nerve growth factor are differentially expressed in adjacent nonneuronal cells of normal and injured tooth pulp. Cell Tissue Res 2000;299(2):225–36.

98. Davidson B, Reich R, Lazarovici P, et al. Expression of the nerve growth factor receptors TrkA and p75 in malignant mesothelioma. Lung Cancer 2004;44(2):159–65.

99. Nie H, Fu Y, Wang CH. Paclitaxel and suramin-loaded core/shell microspheres in the treatment of brain tumors. Biomaterials 2010;31(33):8732–40.

100. Nie H, Dong Z, Arifin DY, et al. Core/shell microspheres via coaxial electrohydrodynamic atomization for sequential and parallel release of drugs. J Biomed Mater Res A 2010;95(3):709–16.

101. Zeng H, Pang X, Wang S, et al. The preparation of core/shell structured microsphere of multi first-line anti-tuberculosis drugs and evaluation of biological safety. Int J Clin Exp Med 2015;8(6):8398–414.

# Regenerative Endodontics by Cell Homing

Ling He, DDS[a,b], Juan Zhong, DDS[a], Qimei Gong, DDS, PhD[a,b],
Bin Cheng, PhD[c,*], Sahng G. Kim, DDS, MS[d,*], Junqi Ling, DDS, PhD[b,*],
Jeremy J. Mao, DDS, PhD[b,e,*]

## KEYWORDS

- Regenerative • Endodontics • Cell homing • Dentin • Dental pulp
- Tissue engineering • Regeneration

## KEY POINTS

- Apical revascularization and platelet-rich plasma are current regenerative treatments for infected immature permanent teeth.
- There are no broadly accepted regenerative therapies for infected dental pulp of mature teeth in adult patients. Two distinctive approaches are being explored: cell transplantation and cell homing.
- Quantitative assessments with proper statistical analyses are required to evaluate the outcome of experimental and clinical studies of pulp regeneration.
- Existing and novel regenerative endodontic therapies may not receive broad clinical adoption without safety and efficacy demonstrated in prospective clinical trials.

## INTRODUCTION

Dental pulp infections resulting from caries or trauma in immature permanent teeth with developing, open root apices represent a formidable clinical challenge. Multiple tooth

Disclosure Statement: The authors have nothing to disclose. Dr J.J. Mao is a founder of Innovative Elements, LLC, which develops regenerative therapies.
[a] Division of Endodontics, Center for Craniofacial Regeneration, Columbia University Medical Center, Columbia University, 630 West 168 Street, New York, NY 10032, USA; [b] Department of Operative Dentistry and Endodontics, Guanghua School of Stomatology, Hospital of Stomatology, Guangdong Province Key Laboratory of Stomatology, Sun Yat-sen University, 56 Lingyuan West Road, Guangzhou, Guangdong, 510055, China; [c] Department of Biostatistics, Columbia University Mailman School of Public Health, 722 West 168th Street, Room 631, New York, NY 10032, USA; [d] Division of Endodontics, Center for Craniofacial Regeneration, Columbia University Medical Center, College of Dental Medicine, Columbia University, 630 West 168 Street - PH7Stem #128, New York, NY 10032, USA; [e] Division of Endodontics, Center for Craniofacial Regeneration, Columbia University Medical Center, Columbia University, 630 West 168 Street - PH7E, New York, NY 10032, USA
* Corresponding author.
E-mail addresses: bc2159@cumc.columbia.edu; sgk2114@columbia.edu; lingjunqi@163.com; jmao@columbia.edu

decays occur among approximately 21% of children from 6 to 11 years of age in the United States, per 2012 Centers for Disease Control and Prevention data.[1] Pulp necrosis rates are as high as 27% among 889 traumatized permanent teeth.[2] Tooth fractures are common among traumatized immature permanent teeth due to thin dentin wall and underdeveloped roots.[3–5] Conventional root canal treatment with gutta-percha is contraindicated for infected immature permanent teeth with open apices.[6] In case of tooth loss, dental implants are further contraindicated in adolescent patients due to submergence of metallic implants in the growing alveolar bone in the vertical dimension.[7] The primary management goal of traumatized and/or infected dental pulp in immature permanent teeth is to control infections, restore dental pulp vitality, and promote the development and maturation of otherwise arrested tooth roots.[8]

The American Association of Endodontists (AAE) has focused its regenerative endodontics effort on revitalization of dental pulp and continuous root development in immature permanent teeth.[9] The American Dental Association (ADA) in 2011 adopted several codes that allow the practice of evoked bleeding or apical revascularization (AR) in infected dental pulp in immature, permanent teeth with traumatic injuries or infections.[10] The AAE's regenerative endodontics initiative has stimulated interest and awareness toward identification of multiple approaches for the restoration of dental pulp in immature permanent teeth with pulp infections.[6,11–13] The current goal of regenerative endodontics is to restore the vitality of dental pulp in immature, developing permanent teeth and to enable otherwise arrested root development.[4,6,11,14,15]

The majority of endodontic patients are adults with well-developed, mature teeth.[16] Each year, approximately 22.3 million endodontic procedures are performed in the United States alone.[17] The most common endodontic treatment in mature teeth is to remove the infected dental pulp, disinfect the root canal, and fill the instrumented root canal with gutta-percha, a bioinert material.[18] During root canal preparation, dentin is ablated by manual or rotary instruments with a conceptual goal to remove bacterial colonies that enter dentinal tubules.[19–21] Conventional endodontic treatments are generally successful and effective in eliminating pain and controlling infections.[22,23] Success and failure rates following root canal treatments performed by general practitioners or endodontists have been documented in clinical outcome studies. Reinfections and tooth fractures are 2 key causes for failure following endodontic treatments.[24–26] One retrospective study revealed a 94.44% overall success rate among 110,766 nonsurgical root canal cases treated by endodontists in a 3.5 year follow-up.[27] However, another study found that success rates for primary root canal treatments were between 68% and 85% in 1-year recall.[23] For primary root canal therapy delivered by general practitioners, approximately 20% of endodontically treated teeth were lost 4 years following treatment.[28] With millions of root canal treatments in the United States per year, and many more worldwide, a double-digit, or even a single-digit, failure rate would mean countless hours of retreatments or tooth loss, representing significant socioeconomic burden for the patient and society.

Regenerative endodontics has been a long-term aspiration to restore the vitality, function, and structure of diseased dental pulp and dentin. However, regenerative endodontic treatments have been applied primarily to immature permanent teeth to date. The term of regenerative endodontics should include revitalization of necrotic immature permanent teeth and mature permanent teeth. Regenerative strategies for infected or traumatized mature permanent teeth in adult patients are being explored as 2 distinctive approaches:

1. Cell transplantation of ex vivo cultivated stem/progenitor cells
2. Cell homing by molecules that recruit the patient's endogenous cells.

In this article, clinical case reports of AR and platelet-rich plasma (PRP) are critically reviewed. It further highlights cell homing as a novel strategy for dental pulp regeneration with potential not only in immature permanent teeth but also in fully mature permanent teeth. It also further benchmarks cell homing with AR and PRP as parallel approaches for regenerative endodontics.

## CHALLENGES AND EFFICACY OF EXISTING REGENERATIVE ENDODONTIC TREATMENTS
### Apical Revascularization or Evoked Bleeding

In 1961, the first case of evoked bleeding in the root canal of immature teeth with pulp necrosis was reported.[29] Microscopic sections obtained from the extracted patient teeth showed ingrowth of fibrous connective tissue in the root canal following evoked bleeding.[29] Over the past approximately 55 years, several experimental studies and isolated clinical cases of AR have been documented. Experimentally, there was ingrowth of connective tissues into root canals of incisors with immature apices in rhesus monkeys following evoked bleeding.[30] Root resorption was noted in some teeth with chronically inflamed granulation tissue.[30] AR applied to 2 clinical cases of immature permanent teeth with chronic apical abscesses and sinus tracts led to apical closure.[31,32] Microscopic images of immature teeth in animal models and isolated clinical cases demonstrate the ingrowth of connective tissue in the root canal, including soft and mineralized tissues,[33–35] with newly formed mineralized tissue characterized as cementum-like or bone-like tissue but not dentin.[35–37] A comprehensive summary of previous clinical case reports of evoked bleeding in immature permanent teeth was provided based on qualitative or semiquantitative outcomes as reported by the original investigators, including apical pathosis, root lengthening, root canal wall thickening, and apical closure.[38] To date, there is no prospective clinical trial on AR.

In 2011, the ADA adopted a procedure code to allow induced apical bleeding into endodontically prepared root canal of immature permanent teeth with necrotic pulp. The ADA procedure includes disinfecting with antibiotics mixture and evoking bleeding from periapical tissue to form blood clot in the root canal as a scaffold for the regeneration of pulp and dentin complex. This ADA procedure is an important step in regenerative endodontics. However, several issues have been identified with the practice of this ADA procedure, including inadequately defined inclusion and exclusion criteria, especially a lack of clear definition on the severity of pulp and/or apical infections; and unclear, nonuniform outcome parameters.[39]

The authors selected a previously published clinical case report[40] for additional analysis. The investigators allocated a total of 20 adolescent and young adult subjects with nonvital, immature permanent teeth for AR or combined AR and PRP (AR + PRP) treatment (10 subjects per group).[40] Multiple strengths of this report[40] include a relatively large sample size (20 subjects in total), reduction in apical radiolucency in most but not all subjects, and long-term follow-up (1 year). In multiple cases, there was calcification bridge formation in the apex, although apical closure was not observed following 1-year follow-up.[40] Only 10 out of the total 20 cases were presented with radiographs in this report: 5 treated with AR and the other 5 treated with AR + PRP.[40] Following medication with triple-antibiotics paste, evoked bleeding was induced in the first group with AR only. The investigators concluded that root length increased following AR treatment (**Table 1**): "+ being satisfactory; ++ being good and +++ being excellent."[40]

Due to the qualitative nature of the investigators' assessment on root lengthening, we measured root lengths before treatment (baseline), at 6-month follow-up, and 12-

**Table 1**
**Radiographic findings at the 1-year follow-up**

| Procedure Performed | Serial Number | Tooth # (Age, Sex) | Radiographic Findings at 1-y Follow-up | | | |
|---|---|---|---|---|---|---|
| | | | Periapical Healing | Apical Closure | Root Lengthening | Dentinal Wall Thickening |
| Revascularization (group 1) (average age = 20.1 y) | 1 | 21 (18 y, F) | ++ | +++ | ++ | ++ |
| | 2 | 21 (16 y, F) | ++ | ++ | ++ | + |
| | 3 | 11 (21 y, M) | + | + | ++ | ++ |
| | 4 | 21 (15 y, M) | ++ | ++ | + | + |
| | 5 | 21 (23 y, M) | ++ | + | ++ | + |
| | 6 | 11 (27 y, M) | ++ | + | + | + |
| | 7 | 11 (18 y, F) | + | + | + | + |
| | 8 | 21 (23 y, F) | + | +++ | ++ | ++ |
| | 9 | 21 (23 y, M) | ++ | ++ | ++ | + |
| | 10 | 21 (17 y, F) | ++ | + | + | + |
| Revascularization + PRP (group 2) (average age = 19.7 y) | 1 | 21 (15 y, M) | ++ | +++ | +++ | ++ |
| | 2 | 11 (21 y, M) | +++ | +++ | ++ | ++ |
| | 3 | 21 (24 y, M) | ++ | +++ | +++ | ++ |
| | 4 | 21 (28 y, F) | ++ | +++ | +++ | +++ |
| | 5 | 21 (15 y, M) | +++ | +++ | ++ | +++ |
| | 6 | 11 (17 y, F) | +++ | ++ | ++ | + |
| | 7 | 21 (22 y, M) | +++ | ++ | ++ | ++ |
| | 8 | 11 (15 y, M) | ++ | +++ | +++ | ++ |
| | 9 | 11 (17 y, F) | +++ | ++ | ++ | + |
| | 10 | 21 (23 y, M) | + | +++ | + | +++ |

*Abbreviations:* F, female; M, male; +, satisfactory; ++, good; +++, excellent.
*From* Jadhav G, Shah N, Logani A. Revascularization with and without platelet-rich plasma in nonvital, immature, anterior teeth: a pilot clinical study. J Endod 2012;38:1586; with permission.

month follow-up (**Fig. 1**). To compensate for frequently unavoidable radiographic distortion with images taken over time, we measured the linear length of not only the treated tooth (TT) but also the adjacent reference tooth (RT) (see **Fig. 1**). We modified a pioneering method to quantitatively measure root length.[41,42] Initially, we measured the linear root length from the apex to the cementoenamel junction (CEJ)[41,42] but encountered the difficulty that it was impossible to visualize CEJ in some teeth due to tooth crowding. Accordingly, all linear measurements were made along the longitudinal axis of the tooth from the apex to incisal edge, with the exception of Case 4A in which the incisal edge of the treated central incisor was cut off in the radiographic image (see **Fig. 1**). To minimize intrinsic radiographic distortion, we further calculated the TT/RT ratio (see **Fig. 1**). All tooth length measurements (treated teeth in red and reference teeth in blue) were overlaid, along with the calculated ratios of the treated versus reference teeth in green. **Fig. 1D** tabulates all tooth length measurements and TT/RT ratios. We uniformly enhanced the contrast of some radiographs to visualize the root apex.

Linear tooth length measurements showed increases in some cases at 6-month and/or 12-month follow-ups. However, the lengths of reference teeth in these subjects also increased (see **Fig. 1**). Importantly, TT/RT ratios showed virtually no increase in tooth lengths (see **Fig. 1D**) by statistical analysis by comparing the ratios of tooth lengths at 12-month follow-up with the baseline before AR treatment (**Fig. 2**), suggesting no increase in tooth length as a result of evoked bleeding or AR treatment. Thus,

# Revascularization Only

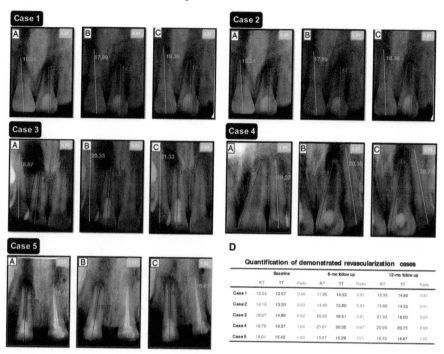

**Fig. 1.** Quantification AR cases. (*A–C*) (Cases 1–5) Tooth length measurements (treated teeth in *red* and reference teeth in *blue*) along the longitudinal axis of the tooth and also the ratio of the treated versus reference teeth in green, with the exception of Case 4A in which the incisal edge of the treated central incisor was cut off the radiographic image. (*D*) All linear measurements of tooth lengths and ratios of treated tooth (TT) and reference tooth (RT) in AR cases. Ratio = TT/RT. (*Adapted from [A–C]* Jadhav G, Shah N, Logani A. Revascularization with and without platelet-rich plasma in nonvital, immature, anterior teeth: a pilot clinical study. J Endod 2012;38:1582–3; with permission.)

this report's conclusion of root length increase[40] following AR treatment seems to be erroneous.

Statistical methods used to calculate the ratios of tooth length measurements in **Fig. 1** and **Fig. 3** are as follows. Due to frequent radiographic image distortion for a given subject taken over time, tooth length ratios were used. The change in tooth length ratios from baseline to 6-month follow-up and 12-month follow-up in AR and AR + PRP groups was compared using a linear mixed-effects model in which treatment, time, and treatment–time interaction were modeled as fixed effects. Random subject effects were included to account for within subject correlations due to repeated measures. A significant interaction effect confirmed the treatment effect. All statistical analysis was conducted in Statistical Analysis System (SAS) version 9.4.

The present quantitative and statistical analysis suggests a need for critical evaluation of published clinical data. A prospective clinical trial with quantitative analysis and statistical power is needed for proper evaluation of the clinical efficacy of AR. Currently, AR is scarcely performed by endodontists in private practice in the United States and even less frequently performed by general dentists. Based on clinical case

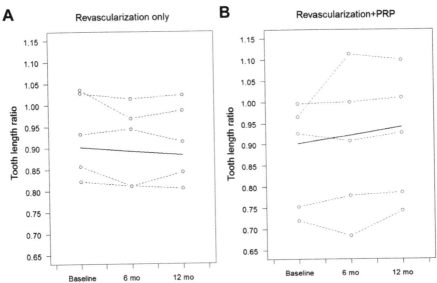

**Fig. 2.** Statistical analysis of quantitated tooth length ratios of demonstrated cases. (*A*) A slight but statistically significant decrease in tooth length ratios at 12-month follow-up in comparison with the baseline (before AR treatment). (*B*) A slight but significant increase in tooth length ratios at 12-month follow-up in comparison with the baseline (before AR + PRP treatment). Furthermore, the AR + PRP group had significantly greater tooth length increase than AR alone (*P* = .039). Dash lines: trend for tooth length ratio of each case; Solid line: Linear trend for root length ratios of all demonstrated cases in each group. (*Data from* Jadhav G, Shah N, Logani A. Revascularization with and without platelet-rich plasma in nonvital, immature, anterior teeth: a pilot clinical study. J Endod 2012;38:1581–7.)

reports, the following challenges have emerged and likely account for scarce clinical acceptance of AR as a regenerative endodontics procedure:

- Inconsistent clinical outcome
- Procedural variation among practitioners
- Interpatient variability of evoked blood clot partially due to different root canal and/or apical pathosis conditions
- Inclusion and exclusion criteria not strictly defined
- Clinical evaluation methods lacking quantitative rigor and/or statistical power
- A lack of prospective clinical trials.

### Platelet-Rich Plasma

PRP is prepared as concentrated platelets from the patient's autologous whole blood.[43] Platelet aggregates harbor approximately 4-fold higher growth factors and cytokines on average than the whole blood.[44] PRP was apparently first used in 1987 in open-heart surgery to avoid excessive blood transfusion.[45] Since then, PRP has been broadly used in many specialties of medicine, including orthopedics[46,47]; ear, nose, and throat[48]; neurosurgery[49]; ophthalmology[50]; urology[51]; wound healing[52]; cosmetic[53]; cardiothoracic[54]; and maxillofacial surgeries.[55] PRP was first used in the oral and dental community along with cancellous bone particulate grafts with a goal to accelerate healing of mandibular continuity defects.[56] Hargreaves and colleagues[57]

# Revascularization + PRP

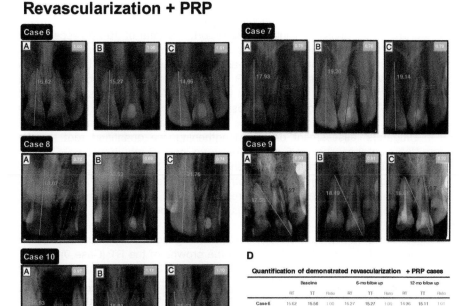

**Fig. 3.** Quantification of demonstrated revascularization + PRP cases. (*A–C*) (Cases 6–10) Tooth length measurements (treated teeth in *red* and reference teeth in *blue*) along the longitudinal axis of the tooth, with the exception of Cases 9 and 10 in which the crowns of the RT (Case 9) and TT (Case 10) were restored and the ratio of the treated versus reference teeth in green of the AR + PRP group. (*D*) All linear measurements of tooth lengths and ratios of TT and RT in revascularization + PRP cases. Ratio = TT/RT. (*Adapted from [A–C]* Jadhav G, Shah N, Logani A. Revascularization with and without platelet-rich plasma in nonvital, immature, anterior teeth: a pilot clinical study. J Endod 2012;38:1584–5; with permission.)

advocated PRP use for regenerative endodontics in 2008. PRP was first attempted as a regenerative endodontics procedure in 2011 in a necrotic, nonvital, immature permanent tooth with an open apex.[58] Following medication with triple-antibiotics paste, PRP was infused into the root canal up to the CEJ.[58] Recall at 5 and one-half months showed apical closure and resolution of periapical lesion, in addition to positive response to both cold tests and electrical pulp testing.[58] In another study, pulp-like connective tissue was present in microscopic sections of extirpated soft tissue 14 months following PRP treatment in the root canal of a nonvital, immature permanent tooth.[59] PRP alone or PRP with transplanted mesenchymal stem/progenitor cells promoted the formation of cementum-like tissue and soft tissue, rather than dentin-like structure, in endodontically prepared root canals in beagle dogs.[60–62] In another study, PRP with or without mesenchymal stem/progenitor cell transplantation showed no significant differences in the amount of soft tissue formation in root canals, nor did PRP show significant differences from the amount of soft tissue formation in root canals by evoked bleeding.[60,63] A clinical case report showed that PRP delivery in the root canal with necrotic pulp in a 39-year-old female subject with extensive periapical radiolucency and open apex yielded resolution of periapical lesion at 30-month follow-up but showed no evidence of root lengthening or thickening.[64]

In the previously analyzed clinical case report,[40] a total of 10 adolescent and young adult subjects with nonvital, immature permanent teeth received PRP treatment. Following medication with triple-antibiotics paste, evoked bleeding was induced, followed by placement of PRP in a collagen sponge in blood evoked from the apex (AR + PRP). Only 5 out of the total 10 AR + PRP cases presented with radiographs in the report.[40] The investigators concluded that root lengthening was observed in the AR + PRP group (see **Table 1**). Due to the qualitative nature of the investigators' assessment on root lengthening, we quantified root lengths before treatment (baseline), at 6-month follow-up, and 12-month follow-up. As for **Fig. 1**, we minimized intrinsic radiographic distortion by calculating the ratio of the TT and adjacent or contralateral tooth as the RT (see **Fig. 3**). **Fig. 3** demonstrates all tooth length measurements (treated teeth in red and reference teeth in blue) and the ratio of the treated versus reference teeth in green of the AR + PRP group.

All linear measurements were made along the longitudinal axis of the tooth, with the exception of Cases 9 and 10 in which the crowns of the RT (Case 9) and TT (Case 10) were restored, following AR + PRP treatment. Statistical analysis revealed a slight but significant increase in the ratio of root lengths at 12-month follow-up in comparison with the baseline (before AR + PRP treatment) (see **Fig. 3**B), primarily owing to Cases 7 and 10, suggesting tooth length increase as a result of combined AR + PRP treatment of 2 out of 5 demonstrated cases and consistent with the investigators' conclusion that PRP may have promoted root lengthening. Furthermore, the change in tooth lengths in the 2 groups had different patterns ($P = .039$). Combined AR + PRP treatment induced a more significant, albeit mild, tooth length increase than AR alone.

Currently, PRP is scarcely adopted by endodontists and even less frequently performed by general dentists in private practice. A prospective clinical trial with quantitative measures and statistical power is needed for proper evaluation of the clinical efficacy of PRP. Multiple retrospective clinical case reports published to date have demonstrated several challenges of PRP use in regenerative endodontic. These challenges have precluded broad acceptance of PRP as a regenerative endodontics procedure:

- Inconsistency in clinical outcome
- Interpractitioner variation owing to different PRP collection methods and concentration of PRP used
- Interpatient variability that is known to be associated with PRP use in other medical fields
- Inclusion and exclusion criteria not well defined
- Clinical evaluation methods lacking quantitative rigor and statistical power
- Lack of prospective clinical trials.

## CELL HOMING

In the context of tissue regeneration, cell homing consists of 2 distinctive cellular processes: recruitment and differentiation. Recruitment refers to directional cell migration, including that of stem/progenitor cells, to the site of tissue defects. Pulp and dentin regeneration will not be possible unless mesenchymal stem/progenitor cells with the capacity to differentiate into multiple cell lineages that form pulp and dentin are recruited into the root canal. Differentiation refers to the process of transformation of stem/progenitor cells into mature cells. In the context of dental pulp and dentin regeneration, stem/progenitor cells differentiate into odontoblasts, pulp fibroblasts, and need to induce the sprouting of neural fibrils and endothelial cells along with other angiogenesis related cells. Whether dental pulp stem/progenitor cells directly differentiate into endothelial cells is an area of meaningful and intense investigations.[65,66]

The concept of cell homing for dental pulp and/or dentin regeneration was introduced in 2010.[67] Growth factors were singularly or in combination delivered into the endodontically prepared root canals of extracted human teeth. All extracted human teeth were sterilized with autoclave to deactivate any remaining proteins in the root canal or dentinal tubules. Collagen gel was infused into endodontically prepared root canals with or without basic fibroblast growth factors (bFGFs), vascular endothelial growth factors (VEGFs), platelet-derived growth factors (PDGFs), nerve growth factors (NGFs), or bone morphogenetic proteins (BMPs) (**Fig. 4**). The treated and control teeth were implanted subcutaneously into Sprague-Dawley rats for 3 to 6 weeks.[67] In vivo harvested samples showed dental pulp–like tissue with blood vessels in endodontically treated root canals as shown in patched multiple histology sections from the root apex to pulp chamber (see **Fig. 4**). We then isolated all the soft tissue in root canals of treated and control human teeth and performed enzyme-linked immunosorbent assay (ELISA) (**Fig. 5**). von Willebrand factor, dentin sialoprotein, and NGF were quantitatively identified following growth factor delivery (see **Fig. 5**), suggesting the presence of blood vessels, dentin-like tissue, and neural-like tissue in regenerated dental pulp in root canals of human teeth on growth factor delivery. No cells were ex vivo cultivated or in vivo transplanted in this study.[67]

Cell homing induced the recruitment of endogenous stem/progenitor cells to the root canal by means such as growth factors, apparently followed by differentiation into dental pulp-like cells (**Fig. 6**). The cell transplantation approach, on the other hand, relies on ex vivo cultivation of stem/progenitor cells that are isolated from the host and transplantation of the cultivated cells into the root canal of the host for pulp and/or dentin regeneration. The cell homing strategy presents a complementary and/or alternative approach to cell transplantation for pulp and/or dentin regeneration.[9,68] Both cell homing and cell transplantation approaches have shown promising outcomes in preclinical animal models for pulp and/or dentin regeneration.[67,69–71] Cell transplantation in dental pulp and/or dentin regeneration is beyond the scope of this article but can be found elsewhere.[70,72–77]

The concept of cell homing in tissue regeneration was first proposed in a *Lancet* report in 2010.[78] The entire articular cartilage layer was regenerated without cell transplantation but, instead, by the delivery of a single growth factor, transforming growth factor-β3 (TGFβ3). Anatomically correct synthetic bioscaffolds designed by 3-dimensional bioprinting technology were used to replace the entire articular surface of humeral condyles of rabbits.[78] The bioscaffolds were not seeded with cells but only embedded with TGFβ3-adsorbed hydrogel.[78] This single growth factor delivery with anatomically precise scaffolds implantation yielded the regeneration of avascular cartilage, which integrated with regenerated vascularized subchondral bone at 4 months postsurgery.[78]

Cell homing with AR and PRP specifically for dental pulp regeneration is benchmarked in (**Table 2**). The comparisons in **Table 2** are debatable. Pain relief and reduction of reinfection have been demonstrated or are probably possible with all 3 approaches, likely attributable primarily to the effectiveness of root canal disinfection. Whereas AR, PRP, and cell homing are all applicable to immature permanent teeth, cell homing may be uniquely suitable for mature permanent teeth (see **Table 2**).

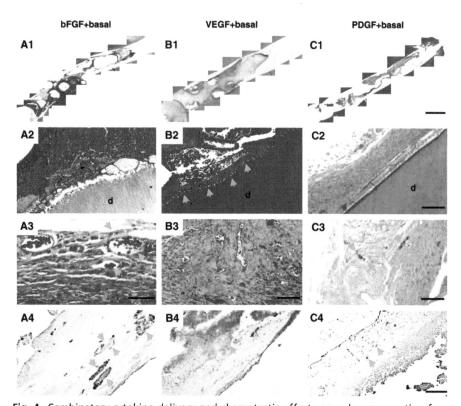

**Fig. 4.** Combinatory cytokine delivery and chemotactic effects on pulp regeneration from host endogenous cells. (*A1*) Combined delivery of basic fibroblast growth factor (bFGF) with basal cytokines of NGF and BMP7 yielded recellularization in the entire endodontically treated root canal as shown by reconstructed, multiple microscopic images from root apex to pulp chamber. (*A2*) Close-up image showing abundant cells and integration with native dentin (d) in endodontically treated root canal. (*A3*) Higher magnification showing erythrocyte-filled blood vessels (*arrows*) in connective tissue. (*A4*) Scattered islands of positive VEGF antibody staining (*arrows*). (*B1*) Combined delivery of VEGF with basal cytokines of NGF and BMP7 induced recellularization in the entire endodontically treated root canal. (*B2*) Connective tissue with abundant cells integrated with native dentin (d), including a layer of dentin-like tissue between abundant cells and dentinal wall (*arrows*). (*B3*) Multiple blood-vessel–like structures in regenerated connective tissue (*arrows*). (*B4*) Positive VEGF antibody staining. Arrows indicate positive VEGF staining. (*C1*) Combined delivery of PDGF with basal cytokines of NGF and BMP7 yielded fully regenerated tissues in the entire endodontically treated root canal. (*C2*) Abundant cells in connective tissue that integrated to native dentin (d). (*C3*) Blood-vessel–like structures (*arrows*) in connective tissue. (*C4*) VEGF antibody staining. Arrows indicate positive VEGF staining. Scale bars (*A1, B1, C1*), 1 mm; (*A2, B2, C2*), 100 μm; (*A3*), 100 μm; (*B3, C3*), 300 μm; and (*A4, B4, C4*), 300 μm. (*From* Kim JY, Xin X, Moioli EK, et al. Regeneration of dental-pulp-like tissue by chemotaxis-induced cell homing. Tissue Eng Part A 2010;16:3026; with permission.)

Although the current focus of regenerative endodontics is to save necrotic immature permanent teeth with open apices, cell homing may be applicable to the restoration of dental pulp vitality of both immature and mature permanent teeth. Almost all AR or PRP studies have been conducted in immature permanent teeth in adolescent and young adult subjects, with several exceptions.[79–82]

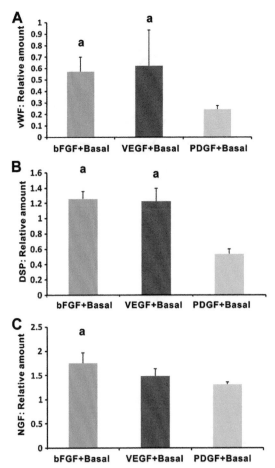

**Fig. 5.** ELISA of von Willebrand factor (vWF), dentin sialoprotein (DSP), and NGF in regenerated dental-pulp-like tissue relative to collagen scaffold only group. (*A*) Codelivery of bFGF or VEGF with basal cytokines of NGF and BMP7 yielded significantly more vWF than PDGF with NGF and BMP7. (*B*) Codelivery of bFGF or VEGF with basal cytokines of NGF and BMP7 yielded significantly more DSP than PDGF with NGF and BMP7. (*C*) Codelivery of bFGF or VEGF with basal cytokines of NGF and BMP7 yielded significantly more NGF than PDGF with NGF and BMP7. $n = 6$; [a] $P<.05$. (*From* Kim JY, Xin X, Moioli EK, et al. Regeneration of dental-pulp-like tissue by chemotaxis-induced cell homing. Tissue Eng Part A 2010;16:3027; with permission.)

Economically, a distinctive advantage of AR is that it does not cost more than the current evoked bleeding procedure itself. PRP involves additional costs, such as the purchase of a PRP machine and consumables with each blood sample, in addition to time spent on blood drawing and PRP preparation. Novel molecules developed for cell homing are consumables with a cost. Procedural and patient variations seem to be intrinsic to AR and PRP. Cell homing uses novel molecules that drive therapeutic efficacy, and may be less sensitive to procedural and patient variations. As point-of-care treatments, AR and PRP will not become an off-the-shelf product. Cell homing is poised to become an off-the-shelf product and, upon proof of safety and efficacy, may be broadly adopted.

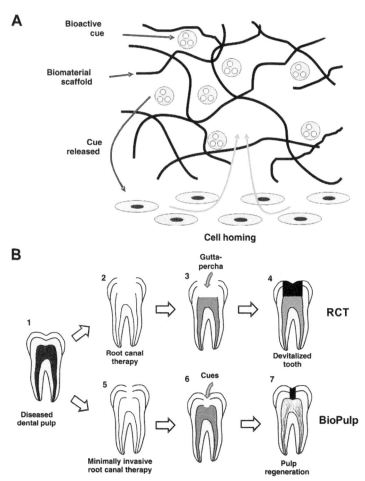

**Fig. 6.** Schemes of cell homing for dental pulp regeneration and clinical translation. (*A*) Bioactive cues can be adsorbed, tethered, or encapsulated in biomaterial scaffolds. On release of bioactive cues, such as from endodontically treated root canals in this work, local and/or systemic cells, including stem/progenitor cells, can be homed in vivo into an anatomic compartment, which, in this case, is root canal that serves as a native scaffold. Current root canal treatment of diseased dental pulp (*B1*) necessitates removal of substantial enamel and dentin structures because obturation of gutta-percha requires unobstructed access (*B2*, *B3*), yet leading to a devitalized tooth (*B4*). The authors propose that a diseased dental pulp (*B1*) can be treated with a revised, minimally invasive root canal therapy (*B5*) on the basis that delivery of injectable bioactive cues does not require unobstructed access to pulp chamber and root canal (*B6*). Although residual inflammation in endodontically treated root canal and periapical region are anticipated to present challenges for pulp regeneration, chemotaxis-induced angiogenesis as shown here may provide the potential for native defense mechanisms that may counteract residue infection in the root canal (*B6*), leading to a vital tooth with regenerated dental pulp (*B7*). (*From* Kim JY, Xin X, Moioli EK, et al. Regeneration of dental-pulp-like tissue by chemotaxis-induced cell homing. Tissue Eng Part A 2010;16:3028; with permission.)

**Table 2**
Benchmarking of apical revascularization, platelet-rich plasma, and cell homing in pulp regeneration

| | Revascularization | PRP | Cell Homing |
|---|---|---|---|
| Relieve pain | √ | √ | √ |
| Prevent reinfection | √ | √ | √ |
| Immature permanent teeth | Yes | Yes | Yes |
| Adult (permanent) teeth | No[79–81] | No[82] | Yes |
| Cost | No | $ | $ |
| Procedural variation | High | High | Low |
| Patient variation | High | High | Low |
| Off-the-shelf product | No | No | Yes |

## SUMMARY

AR and PRP are 2 existing regenerative endodontic treatments. Over the past 55 years, dating back to 1961, AR has been reported in hundreds of clinical case reports but no prospective clinical trial has been conducted to fully understand its safety and efficacy. In isolated clinical cases, there is no question that certainly teeth following AR treatment have completed apical closure and become absent of pretreatment apical radiolucency. However, the clinical outcome of AR has been variable and inconsistent. PRP was first used as a regenerative endodontic treatment in 2011. In multiple preclinical animal studies and isolated clinical case reports, PRP induced ingrowth of vascularized connective tissue in endodontically disinfected root canals but with little evidence of dentin formation. Similar to AR, there has been no prospective clinical trial for PRP. Cell homing has the advantage to the patient's own recruit mesenchymal stem/progenitor cells into endodontically prepared root canals and induce them to differentiate along pulp cell and/or odontoblastic lineages. Different cell homing molecules may be tailored for these purposes. Dispassionate debate in the community and properly designed prospective clinical trials are necessary to identify indications and contraindications of AR, PRP, and cell homing. Regenerative endodontics should encompass both immature permanent teeth and adult (permanent) teeth, especially in consideration of cell homing and cell transplantation as new, putative regenerative approaches for pulp and/or dentin regeneration. Multiple therapeutic approaches should be developed for infected dental pulp of immature and mature permanent teeth, just as multiple drugs are needed for hypertension.

## ACKNOWLEDGMENTS

We thank Drs Lusai Xiang, Jinxuan Zheng, Mo Chen, Yongxing Liu, Xuguang Nie, Xi Wei, Jiayuan Wu and Hanying Bai for scientific discussion, and Ms F. Guo, Y.W. Tse and P. Ralph-Birkett for their administrative assistance. The work is supported by NIH grants R01DE023112, R01DE025643 and R01AR065023 to J.J. Mao, Guangdong Pioneer Grant (52000-52010002) and Guangdong Science and Technology Program (2016B030229003).

## REFERENCES

1. Available at: http://www.cdc.gov/nchs/data/databriefs/db191.htm. Accessed April 18, 2016.

2. Hecova H, Tzigkounakis V, Merglova V, et al. A retrospective study of 889 injured permanent teeth. Dent Traumatol 2010;26:466–75.

3. Andreasen JO, Ravn JJ. Epidemiology of traumatic dental injuries to primary and permanent teeth in a Danish population sample. Int J Oral Surg 1972;1:235–9.

4. Hargreaves KM, Diogenes A, Teixeira FB. Treatment options: biological basis of regenerative endodontic procedures. Pediatr Dent 2013;35:129–40.

5. Shah N, Logani A, Bhaskar U, et al. Efficacy of revascularization to induce apexification/apexogensis in infected, nonvital, immature teeth: a pilot clinical study. J Endod 2008;34:919–25 [discussion: 1157].

6. Garcia-Godoy F, Murray PE. Recommendations for using regenerative endodontic procedures in permanent immature traumatized teeth. Dent Traumatol 2012;28:33–41.

7. Op Heij DG, Opdebeeck H, van Steenberghe D, et al. Age as compromising factor for implant insertion. Periodontol 2000 2003;33:172–84.

8. American Academy on Pediatric Dentistry Clinical Affairs Committee-Pulp Therapy subcommittee, American Academy on Pediatric Dentistry Council on Clinical Affairs. Guideline on pulp therapy for primary and young permanent teeth. Pediatr Dent 2008;30:170–4.

9. Mao JJ, Kim SG, Zhou J, et al. Regenerative endodontics: barriers and strategies for clinical translation. Dent Clin North Am 2012;56:639–49.

10. Available at: http://www.aae.org/regeneration/. Accessed April 18, 2016.

11. Law AS. Considerations for regeneration procedures. Pediatr Dent 2013;35:141–52.

12. Huang GT. Pulp and dentin tissue engineering and regeneration: current progress. Regen Med 2009;4:697–707.

13. Huang GT. The coming era of regenerative endodontics: what an endodontist needs to know. Alpha Omegan 2011;104:46–51.

14. Simon S, Smith AJ. Regenerative endodontics. Br Dent J 2014;216:E13.

15. Goodis HE, Kinaia BM, Kinaia AM, et al. Regenerative endodontics and tissue engineering: what the future holds? Dent Clin North Am 2012;56:677–89.

16. Ingle's Endodontics, fourth edition. Chapter 1, page 3–4.

17. Available at: http://www.aae.org/about-aae/news-room/endodontic-treatment-statistics.aspx. Accessed April 18, 2016.

18. Carrotte P. Endodontics: Part 5. Basic instruments and materials for root canal treatment. Br Dent J 2004;197:455–64 [quiz: 505].

19. Al-Nazhan S, Al-Sulaiman A, Al-Rasheed F, et al. Microorganism penetration in dentinal tubules of instrumented and retreated root canal walls. In vitro SEM study. Restor Dent Endod 2014;39:258–64.

20. Violich DR, Chandler NP. The smear layer in endodontics - a review. Int Endod J 2010;43:2–15.

21. Peters LB, Wesselink PR, Buijs JF, et al. Viable bacteria in root dentinal tubules of teeth with apical periodontitis. J Endod 2001;27:76–81.

22. Ng YL, Mann V, Rahbaran S, et al. Outcome of primary root canal treatment: systematic review of the literature – Part 2. Influence of clinical factors. Int Endod J 2008;41:6–31.

23. Ng YL, Mann V, Rahbaran S, et al. Outcome of primary root canal treatment: systematic review of the literature - part 1. Effects of study characteristics on probability of success. Int Endod J 2007;40:921–39.

24. Akbar I. Radiographic study of the problems and failures of endodontic treatment. Int J Health Sci (Qassim) 2015;9:111–8.

25. Rafter M. Endodontic retreatment: evaluating success and dealing with failures. J Ir Dent Assoc 2003;49:3–8, 10-12, 14.

26. Caliskan MK, Kaval ME, Tekin U, et al. Radiographic and histological evaluation of persistent periapical lesions associated with endodontic failures after apical microsurgery. Int Endod J 2015;48:815–910.

27. Lazarski MP, Walker WA 3rd, Flores CM, et al. Epidemiological evaluation of the outcomes of nonsurgical root canal treatment in a large cohort of insured dental patients. J Endod 2001;27:791–6.

28. Fonzar F, Fonzar A, Buttolo P, et al. The prognosis of root canal therapy: a 10-year retrospective cohort study on 411 patients with 1175 endodontically treated teeth. Eur J Oral Implantol 2009;2:201–8.

29. Ostby BN. The role of the blood clot in endodontic therapy. An experimental histologic study. Acta Odontol Scand 1961;19:324–53.

30. Myers WC, Fountain SB. Dental pulp regeneration aided by blood and blood substitutes after experimentally induced periapical infection. Oral Surg Oral Med Oral Pathol 1974;37:441–50.

31. Iwaya SI, Ikawa M, Kubota M. Revascularization of an immature permanent tooth with apical periodontitis and sinus tract. Dent Traumatol 2001;17:185–7.

32. Banchs F, Trope M. Revascularization of immature permanent teeth with apical periodontitis: new treatment protocol? J Endod 2004;30:196–200.

33. Thibodeau B, Teixeira F, Yamauchi M, et al. Pulp revascularization of immature dog teeth with apical periodontitis. J Endod 2007;33:680–9.

34. Zhu X, Wang Y, Liu Y, et al. Immunohistochemical and histochemical analysis of newly formed tissues in root canal space transplanted with dental pulp stem cells plus platelet-rich plasma. J Endod 2014;40:1573–8.

35. Wang X, Thibodeau B, Trope M, et al. Histologic characterization of regenerated tissues in canal space after the revitalization/revascularization procedure of immature dog teeth with apical periodontitis. J Endod 2010;36:56–63.

36. Shimizu E, Jong G, Partridge N, et al. Histologic observation of a human immature permanent tooth with irreversible pulpitis after revascularization/regeneration procedure. J Endod 2012;38:1293–7.

37. Diogenes A, Ruparel NB, Shiloah Y, et al. Regenerative endodontics: a way forward. J Am Dent Assoc 2016;147:372–80.

38. Law AS. Considerations for regeneration procedures. J Endod 2013;39:S44–56.

39. Lin LM, Ricucci D, Huang GT. Regeneration of the dentine-pulp complex with revitalization/revascularization therapy: challenges and hopes. Int Endod J 2014;47:713–24.

40. Jadhav G, Shah N, Logani A. Revascularization with and without platelet-rich plasma in nonvital, immature, anterior teeth: a pilot clinical study. J Endod 2012;38:1581–7.

41. Bose R, Nummikoski P, Hargreaves K. A retrospective evaluation of radiographic outcomes in immature teeth with necrotic root canal systems treated with regenerative endodontic procedures. J Endod 2009;35:1343–9.

42. Nagy MM, Tawfik HE, Hashem AA, et al. Regenerative potential of immature permanent teeth with necrotic pulps after different regenerative protocols. J Endod 2014;40:192–8.

43. Marx RE. Platelet-rich plasma (PRP): what is PRP and what is not PRP? Implant Dent 2001;10:225–8.

44. Platelet-Rich Plasma, Regenerative Medicine: Sports Medicine, Orthopedic, and Recovery of Musculoskeletal Injuries. Chapter 1, Page 8–9.

45. Ferrari M, Zia S, Valbonesi M, et al. A new technique for hemodilution, preparation of autologous platelet-rich plasma and intraoperative blood salvage in cardiac surgery. Int J Artif Organs 1987;10:47–50.

46. Alsousou J, Thompson M, Hulley P, et al. The biology of platelet-rich plasma and its application in trauma and orthopaedic surgery: a review of the literature. J Bone Joint Surg Br 2009;91:987–96.

47. McCarrel TM, Mall NA, Lee AS, et al. Considerations for the use of platelet-rich plasma in orthopedics. Sports Med 2014;44:1025–36.

48. Rice DH. Platelet-rich plasma in endoscopic sinus surgery. Ear Nose Throat J 2006;85:516, 518.

49. Emel E, Ergun SS, Kotan D, et al. Effects of insulin-like growth factor-I and platelet-rich plasma on sciatic nerve crush injury in a rat model. J Neurosurg 2011;114:522–8.

50. Alio JL, Arnalich-Montiel F, Rodriguez AE. The role of "eye platelet rich plasma" (E-PRP) for wound healing in ophthalmology. Curr Pharm Biotechnol 2012;13:1257–65.

51. Shirvan MK, Alamdari DH, Ghoreifi A. A novel method for iatrogenic vesicovaginal fistula treatment: autologous platelet rich plasma injection and platelet rich fibrin glue interposition. J Urol 2013;189:2125–9.

52. Massara M, Barilla D, De Caridi G, et al. Application of autologous platelet-rich plasma to enhance wound healing after lower limb revascularization: A case series and literature review. Semin Vasc Surg 2015;28:195–200.

53. Kalyam K, Kavoussi SC, Ehrlich M, et al. Irreversible blindness following periocular autologous platelet-rich plasma skin rejuvenation treatment. Ophthal Plast Reconstr Surg 2016;32:79–159.

54. Patel AN, Selzman CH, Kumpati GS, et al. Evaluation of autologous platelet rich plasma for cardiac surgery: outcome analysis of 2000 patients. J Cardiothorac Surg 2016;11:62.

55. Hatakeyama I, Marukawa E, Takahashi Y, et al. Effects of platelet-poor plasma, platelet-rich plasma, and platelet-rich fibrin on healing of extraction sockets with buccal dehiscence in dogs. Tissue Eng Part A 2014;20:874–82.

56. Whitman DH, Berry RL, Green DM. Platelet gel: an autologous alternative to fibrin glue with applications in oral and maxillofacial surgery. J Oral Maxillofac Surg 1997;55:1294–9.

57. Hargreaves KM, Geisler T, Henry M, et al. Regeneration potential of the young permanent tooth: what does the future hold? Pediatr Dent 2008;30:253–60.

58. Torabinejad M, Turman M. Revitalization of tooth with necrotic pulp and open apex by using platelet-rich plasma: a case report. J Endod 2011;37:265–8.

59. Torabinejad M, Faras H. A clinical and histological report of a tooth with an open apex treated with regenerative endodontics using platelet-rich plasma. J Endod 2012;38:864–8.

60. Zhu W, Zhu X, Huang GT, et al. Regeneration of dental pulp tissue in immature teeth with apical periodontitis using platelet-rich plasma and dental pulp cells. Int Endod J 2013;46:962–70.

61. Del Fabbro M, Lolato A, Bucchi C, et al. Autologous Platelet Concentrates for Pulp and Dentin Regeneration: A Literature Review of Animal Studies. J Endod 2016;42:250–7.

62. Torabinejad M, Faras H, Corr R, et al. Histologic examinations of teeth treated with 2 scaffolds: a pilot animal investigation. J Endod 2014;40:515–20.

63. Torabinejad M, Milan M, Shabahang S, et al. Histologic examination of teeth with necrotic pulps and periapical lesions treated with 2 scaffolds: an animal investigation. J Endod 2015;41:846–52.

64. Wang Y, Zhu X, Zhang C. Pulp Revascularization on Permanent Teeth with Open Apices in a Middle-aged Patient. J Endod 2015;41:1571–5.
65. Rosa V, Botero TM, Nor JE. Regenerative endodontics in light of the stem cell paradigm. Int Dent J 2011;61(Suppl 1):23–8.
66. Casagrande L, Cordeiro MM, Nor SA, et al. Dental pulp stem cells in regenerative dentistry. Odontology 2011;99:1–7.
67. Kim JY, Xin X, Moioli EK, et al. Regeneration of dental-pulp-like tissue by chemotaxis-induced cell homing. Tissue Eng Part A 2010;16:3023–31.
68. Kim SG, Zheng Y, Zhou J, et al. Dentin and dental pulp regeneration by the patient's endogenous cells. Endod Topics 2013;28:106–17.
69. Ishizaka R, Iohara K, Murakami M, et al. Regeneration of dental pulp following pulpectomy by fractionated stem/progenitor cells from bone marrow and adipose tissue. Biomaterials 2012;33:2109–18.
70. Iohara K, Imabayashi K, Ishizaka R, et al. Complete pulp regeneration after pulpectomy by transplantation of CD105+ stem cells with stromal cell-derived factor-1. Tissue Eng Part A 2011;17:1911–20.
71. Iohara K, Zheng L, Ito M, et al. Regeneration of dental pulp after pulpotomy by transplantation of CD31(-)/CD146(-) side population cells from a canine tooth. Regen Med 2009;4:377–85.
72. Iohara K, Murakami M, Takeuchi N, et al. A novel combinatorial therapy with pulp stem cells and granulocyte colony-stimulating factor for total pulp regeneration. Stem Cells Transl Med 2013;2:521–33.
73. Caton J, Bostanci N, Remboutsika E, et al. Future dentistry: cell therapy meets tooth and periodontal repair and regeneration. J Cell Mol Med 2011;15:1054–65.
74. Huang GT, Yamaza T, Shea LD, et al. Stem/progenitor cell-mediated de novo regeneration of dental pulp with newly deposited continuous layer of dentin in an in vivo model. Tissue Eng Part A 2010;16:605–15.
75. Nakashima M, Iohara K, Sugiyama M. Human dental pulp stem cells with highly angiogenic and neurogenic potential for possible use in pulp regeneration. Cytokine Growth Factor Rev 2009;20:435–40.
76. Huang GT, Gronthos S, Shi S. Mesenchymal stem cells derived from dental tissues vs. those from other sources: their biology and role in regenerative medicine. J Dent Res 2009;88:792–806.
77. Nakashima M, Iohara K. Mobilized dental pulp stem cells for pulp regeneration: initiation of clinical trial. J Endod 2014;40:S26–32.
78. Lee CH, Cook JL, Mendelson A, et al. Regeneration of the articular surface of the rabbit synovial joint by cell homing: a proof of concept study. Lancet 2010;376:440–8.
79. Saoud TM, Martin G, Chen YH, et al. Treatment of mature permanent teeth with necrotic pulps and apical periodontitis using regenerative endodontic procedures: a case series. J Endod 2016;42:57–65.
80. Shah N, Logani A. SealBio: A novel, non-obturation endodontic treatment based on concept of regeneration. J Conserv Dent 2012;15:328–32.
81. Paryani K, Kim SG. Regenerative endodontic treatment of permanent teeth after completion of root development: a report of 2 cases. J Endod 2013;39:929–34.
82. Priya MH, Tambakad PB, Naidu J. Pulp and periodontal regeneration of an avulsed permanent mature incisor using platelet-rich plasma after delayed replantation: a 12-month clinical case study. J Endod 2016;42:66–71.

# Mesenchymal Stem Cells and Their Role in Dental Medicine

Xueli Mao, DDS, PhD[a,b], Yao Liu, DDS, PhD[a,c], Chider Chen, PhD[a],
Songtao Shi, DDS, PhD[a],*

## KEYWORDS

- Mesenchymal stem cells • Dental stem cell • Cell therapy • Tissue regeneration
- Immunomodulation

## KEY POINTS

- Orofacial/dental tissue contains multiple types of mesenchymal stem cells, including dental pulp stem cells, stem cells from human exfoliated deciduous teeth, periodontal ligament stem cells, stem cells from apical papilla, dental follicle precursor cells, and gingival mesenchymal stem cells.
- These mesenchymal stem cells are capable of regenerating mineralized and nonmineralized orofacial/dental tissues, such as dental pulp and periodontal tissue.
- These mesenchymal stem cells are able to regulate immune response and thus treat a variety of autoimmune diseases.

## INTRODUCTION

In mammals, there are 2 types of stem cells: embryonic stem (ES) cells from the inner cell mass of blastocysts and adult stem cells from adult tissues. Recently, another type of nonembryonic stem cells, known as induced pluripotent stem cells, was isolated. These somatic cells are reprogramed by defined transcription factors to generate ES cell–like cells.[1] ES cells can differentiate into 3 germ layers and adult stem cells are limited to differentiate into distinct cell types. Although ES cells have greater potential to be used for tissue regeneration than adult stem cells, several ethical and legal controversies still hamper their clinical application. The primary role of adult stem cells is to maintain and repair the tissue in which they reside.

[a] Department of Anatomy and Cell Biology, School of Dental Medicine, University of Pennsylvania, Philadelphia, PA, USA; [b] Department of Operative Dentistry and Endodontics, Guanghua School of Stomatology, Affiliated Stomatological Hospital, Sun Yat-sen University, 55 West Lingyuan Rd, Yuexiu District, Guangzhou 510055, China; [c] Department of Pediatric Dentistry, School of Stomatology, China Medical University, 117 South Nanjing Street, Heping District, Shenyang 110002, China
* Corresponding author. Department of Anatomy and Cell Biology, School of Dental Medicine, University of Pennsylvania, 240 South 40th Street, 420 Levy BLDG, Philadelphia, PA 19104-6004.
*E-mail address:* songtaos@dental.upenn.edu

Dent Clin N Am 61 (2017) 161–172
http://dx.doi.org/10.1016/j.cden.2016.08.006
0011-8532/17/© 2016 Elsevier Inc. All rights reserved.
dental.theclinics.com

They are currently the most commonly used cell source for clinical therapies. Depending on intrinsic signals modulated by extracellular factors in the stem cell niche, these cells may undergo either prolonged self-renewal or differentiation. In recent years, stem cells have drawn great attention from researchers and clinicians for tissue regeneration and systemic disease treatment.

## MESENCHYMAL STEM CELLS IN OROFACIAL TISSUE

One type of adult stem cells, mesenchymal stem cells (MSCs), was first identified and isolated from bone marrow as an adherent fibroblastlike population with a capacity to differentiate into cells of various lineages.[2] Although bone marrow MSCs (BMMSCs) have been recognized as the classic and principal source of MSCs for most scientific investigations and preclinical studies, non–marrow tissue-derived MSCs were identified in almost all tissues, including placenta, umbilical cord blood, adipose tissue, dermis, and orofacial tissue.[3] During embryonic development, MSCs arise from 2 major sources: neural crest and mesoderm. Craniofacial-derived MSCs are commonly considered to be of neural crest origin, whereas nonorofacial MSCs are mainly derived from mesoderm.[4–6] MSCs derived from different sources have been reported to vary in their proliferative and multilineage differentiation potential, which may contribute to differential roles in regenerative medicine. The abilities of self-renewal and differentiation along various cell lineages make orofacial MSCs an ideal candidate for tissue regeneration. MSCs derived from orofacial tissues are attractive postnatal stem cells for hard tissue regeneration, based on their superior osteogenic properties compared with BMMSCs. In addition, the neural crest origin of orofacial MSCs makes them well suited for regeneration of neural crest–derived craniofacial tissue.[7] Recently, several groups have developed new insight into the immunomodulatory properties of MSCs, which can be exploited to treat systemic immune diseases.[3] Craniofacial MSCs have been identified as a promising cell source with strong immune suppressive ability in systemic immunity to treat autoimmune diseases because of their unique biological characteristics.[8]

### Definition of Mesenchymal Stem Cells

Because several cell populations with similar characteristics and multipotent lineage differentiation potential have been successfully identified in many adult and fetal tissues in addition to bone marrow, MSCs have been used to describe almost all the progenitor cells with multilineage differentiation potential from these parenchymal nonhematopoietic tissues. Although there are currently no unique markers to exclusively identify and characterize MSCs, it is still necessary to propose criteria to define MSCs for both laboratory-based scientific investigations and preclinical studies. First, MSCs are plastic adherent and referred to as colony-forming unit fibroblasts (CFU-f) when maintained in standard culture conditions using tissue culture flasks. Second, MSC populations express stromal markers cluster of differentiation (CD105), CD73, and CD90, but lack the expression of CD45, CD34, CD14, CD11b, CD79a, or CD19 and human leukocyte antigen - antigen D related (HLA-DR) surface markers. Third, the cells must be able to differentiate into osteoblasts, adipocytes, and chondrocytes under defined in vitro differentiating conditions.[9]

### Biological Properties of Mesenchymal Stem Cells

MSCs are nurtured in specialized but poorly identified niche areas by interacting with extracellular matrix (ECM), soluble factors, and surrounding cells, which together regulate the size of stem cell pool and lineage selection by switching MSCs between symmetric and asymmetric cell divisions. Mitotic division of MSC gives rise to 2 cells in symmetric or asymmetric mode. Autologous MSCs from various sources in adults are able to expand MSC numbers to replace the original stem cells for self-renewal via symmetric cell division. Under specific stimulation, MSCs have the potential to generate progenitor cells that are responsible for the production of differentiated cell types in tissue. The balance of MSC division is controlled by developmental and environmental signals to produce an appropriate number of stem cells and differentiated cells.[10] It is well known that differentiated cells have a limited proliferative capacity caused by the loss of telomere length after each mitotic division. Because MSCs express telomerase and maintain longer telomeres than other somatic cells, they have enormous proliferative capacities. As a result, MSCs are able to extend more than 10 passages in vitro without losing their original characteristics.[11,12] Under culture conditions containing specific growth factors and chemical reagents, MSCs are able to differentiate into multilineage cell types of endodermal, ectodermal, and mesodermal origins, including osteocytes, chondrocytes, endothelial cells, adipocytes, myocytes, cardiomyocytes, neuronal cells, and hepatocytes.[13] Thus, MSCs have been identified as a significant cell source for regenerative medicine.

In addition to generating structures to replace damaged and diseased tissues, in the past decade, another unique property of MSCs has been discovered: that they have profound immunomodulatory functions. MSCs are able to interplay with several types of immune cells, including T lymphocytes, B lymphocytes, natural killer (NK) cells, and dendritic cells (DCs). Numerous studies have reported that MSCs induce immune cell apoptosis and inhibit immune cell proliferation by means of direct cell-cell contact and soluble antiinflammatory factor secretion.[14] T cells play an important role in the adaptive immune system. It has been shown that MSCs efficiently suppress proliferation of $CD4^+$ T cells by arresting them in the G0/G1 phase.[15] Moreover, MSCs are able to reduce production of interferon gamma (IFN-$\gamma$) from T-helper (Th) 1 cells and interleukin (IL)-17 from Th17 cells.[16,17] Regulatory T cells (Tregs) are a functionally distinct $CD4^+$ T-cell population in the peripheral blood that suppresses autoimmune response.[18] MSCs have been reported to directly or indirectly promote the proliferation of Tregs and enhance their regulatory capacity.[19] Systemic MSC administration has been used to treat a variety of autoimmune diseases. However, the detailed mechanism in which a single shot of MSCs provides long-lasting amelioration of the autoimmune environment is not fully understood. Instead of engraftment to defect organs, systemic infusion of MSCs induces a transient T-cell apoptosis via the Fas ligand (FasL)–mediated Fas death pathway and ameliorates diseased phenotypes in autoimmune systemic sclerosis/scleroderma and colitis mouse models. The therapeutic mechanism of MSC infusion is associated with phagocytosis of apoptotic T-cell debris, leading to a high level of macrophage-mediated transforming growth factor beta (TGF$\beta$) production and a subsequent immune tolerance for immunotherapy by regulatory T cell (Treg) upregulation. In addition, mechanistic study shows that Fas governs monocyte chemotactic protein-1 secretion in MSCs, which plays a crucial role in the recruitment of T cells to MSCs for FasL-mediated apoptosis.[20] Therefore, MSCs have been regarded as strong candidates for clinical application in the treatment of immune disorders. These immunomodulatory properties are not only specific to MSCs from bone marrow but also are inherent to MSCs from the orofacial region.

## Dental Tissue Derived Mesenchymal Stem Cell

Dental tissue is a specialized tissue that does not show continuous remodeling like bony tissue. Nonetheless, it has been reported that dental tissue–derived MSC-like populations have been isolated and characterized. Dental stem cells were first isolated from human pulp tissue and were termed postnatal dental pulp stem cells (DPSCs).[21] DPSCs isolated from enzymatic treatment of human dental pulp tissue are able to form

CFU-f with various characteristics, suggesting heterogeneity.[22,23] These cells have the capacity for multilineage differentiation even if they seem to be more committed to odontogenic rather than osteogenic differentiation, with specific dentinlike structure formation.[24] Compared with BMMSCs, multiple colony-derived DPSCs show a higher in vitro proliferation capability that could vary from 60 to 120 population doublings before showing signs of cell senescence.[21] Note that dental mesenchyme is usually termed ectomesenchyme because of its earlier interaction with the neural crest, during embryonic development. Thus, ectomesenchyme-derived dental stem cells may possess different characteristics akin to those of neural crest cells. From this prospective, successive isolation of MSC-like cells from human exfoliated deciduous teeth (SHED) seems to be of particular interest. SHED also showed the ability to differentiate into adipogenic, osteogenic, myogenic, and chondrogenic lineages.[25,26] In addition, under neurogenic conditions, SHEDs show multicytoplasmic processes instead of the typical fibroblastic morphology while increasing the expression of neural markers, such as βIII-tubulin, glutamic acid decarboxylase (GAD), and neuronal nuclei (NeuN).[25] Moreover, SHED have higher expansion potential compared with DPSCs and BMMSCs, reaching around 140 population doublings. Subsequently, 5 more types of dental MSC-like populations have been isolated and characterized: stem cells from periodontal ligament stem cells (PDLSCs),[27] apical papilla (SCAP),[28] dental follicle precursor cells,[29] MSCs from gingiva (GMSCs),[30] and orofacial bone/bone marrow-derived MSCs (OMSCs).[31] However, the precise relationships among these cell populations need to be more extensively investigated.

During the characterization of these dental stem cells, certain aspects of their properties have been compared with those of BMMSCs. Although DPSCs and BMMSCs are regulated by similar factors, and share a common protein expression profile, these populations differ significantly in their proliferative ability and multilineage differentiation potential in vitro, and more importantly in their ability to develop into distinct tissues representative of the microenvironments from which they were derived in vivo. BMMSCs formed only bone tissue in the nude mice model, whereas DPSCs were able to form dentin-pulp structure, although treated in a similar manner. The chondrogenic potential of DPSCs is weak, and the adipogenic potentials of DPSCs and SCAP are weaker compared with BMMSCs.[28,32] In contrast, the neurogenicity of dental stem cells is more potent than BMMSCs, most probably because of their neural crest origin. Dental tissue–derived MSCs have higher a proliferation rate than BMMSCs. For clinical applications, these dental stem cells could be cultured and expanded to obtain a sufficient number of cells, so they represent an accessible and promising resource for MSC-based cell therapy.

Many in vivo and in vitro studies have reported that MSCs from orofacial regions, including DPSCs, SHED, PDLSC, SCAP, GMSCs, and OMSCs, have similar immunomodulation properties to MSCs from bone marrow. DPSCs showed 91.4% inhibition of phytohaemagglutinin (PHA)-activated T-cell response as assessed by a 3H-thymidine assay in a coculture system.[33] SHED can inhibit secretion of IL-17 in vitro, and they are capable of effectively reversing disease phenotype in systemic lupus erythematosus (SLE)–associated MRL/lpr mice and acute colitis mice by increasing the ratio of Tregs to Th17 cells.[8,34] Recently, systemic infusion of SHED successfully ameliorate osteoporotic phenotype by reducing Th1 and Th17 levels in the recipient ovariectomy mice, suggesting that orofacial-derived stem cells are an appropriate cell source for rescuing the estrogen-deficient osteoporosis by rebuilding the recipients' immune homeostasis.[35] GMSCs suppressed peripheral blood lymphocyte proliferation, and induced expression of a wide panel of immunosuppressive factors, including IL-10, indoleamine 2,3-dioxygenase (IDO), inducible nitric oxide synthase, and cyclooxygenase-2.[30] In addition, it has been found that around 90% of GMSCs are derived from neural crest origins, and these show superior effects in ameliorating the inflammatory-related disease phenotype in mice with acute colitis.[36] Other dental stem cells, including SCAP, PDLSCs, and OMSCs, also showed immunosuppressive properties in vitro.[31,37,38]

## DENTAL MESENCHYMAL STEM CELL–BASED THERAPIES FOR REGENERATIVE MEDICINE

Repair and reconstruction of damaged craniofacial tissues are challenging clinical situations because the craniofacial region is a complex construct, consisting of bone, cartilage, ligamentous tissue, soft tissue, and neurovascular bundles. Stem cell–based tissue engineering using MSCs has been considered a promising mode in regenerative medicine.[39–41] Dental stem cells have high proliferation rates and are capable of forming specialized dental tissues. Animal research has proved its feasibility to regenerate these tissues/organs, and clinical trials were also performed.

### Biotooth/Bioroot Engineering

Dental implants are the most suitable clinical treatment of the missing teeth, but they do not integrate into the alveolar bone and connect with a natural periodontal ligament. Developing a fully functioning bioengineered root is the ultimate goal of tooth regeneration. Building an entire tooth logically may require the cooperation of all cell types isolated from tooth buds and a suitable biological scaffold. The recombination of dissociated dental epithelial stem cells and MSCs has been tested on ectopic tooth formation in vivo. The bioengineered teeth produced in ectopic sites grew without some essential elements, such as the complete root and periodontal tissues that allow correct anchoring into the alveolar bone.[42,43]

Instead of attempting to form a whole tooth, a functional bioroot structure for artificial crown restoration has been proved to be practical, by using allogeneic dental tissue–derived MSCs. A mini-swine model was used, and autologous SCAP and PDLSCs were loaded onto hydroxyapatite/tricalcium phosphate (HA/TCP) and Gelfoam scaffolds, respectively, and implanted into sockets of the lower jaw. Three months later, the bioroot structure composed of dentin was randomly deposited by the SCAP. The bioroot was encircled with periodontal ligament tissue and appeared to have a natural relationship with the surrounding bone.[44,45] It should be emphasized that mechanical force is essential for the reconstruction of periodontal ligament–like tissue. These studies suggest a future application of stem cell therapy in tooth/root regeneration.

### Regeneration of Periodontal Defects

It has been shown that stem cell–based periodontal regeneration is most likely to produce reliable and effective results in the management of periodontal defects, particularly of the large tissue defects caused by the disease. PDLSCs, isolated from periodontal ligament, may be the first candidate cellular source for regeneration of periodontal defects. A cementum/periodontal ligament–like structure was regenerated with PDLSC transplant into nude mice.[27] Several researches have investigated the potential use of PDLSCs to treat periodontal diseases in larger animal models and clinical trials.[46,47] Pilot studies have shown efficacy after transplant of periodontal ligament cell sheets, which were able to regenerate periodontal tissue in experimental disease models in rats, dogs, and swine. Clinical studies in human have shown that using autologous PDLSCs to treat periodontal intrabony defects was safe and showed a significant increase in the alveolar bone height or decrease in the bone defect depth over time.[47]

In recent years, cell sheet engineering without a scaffold for regeneration of peri-odontal tissues has received increased attention. The continuous cell sheet not only provides sufficient PDLSCs physically but also prevents degradation of the deposited ECM caused by enzymes. PDLSC cell sheet serves as a three-dimensional substruc-ture for cell adhesion and also acts as a reservoir for growth factors and signals for specialized differentiation. Cell sheets of human PDLSCs have been successfully created. Cementum/periodontal ligament complexes have been observed by trans-planting layered PDLSCs sheets in vivo.[48,49] Moreover, a clinical study using PDLSCs for periodontal regeneration in humans was also based on cell sheet delivery, which suggested that this technique was a clinically translatable approach.[50] However, the safety of PDLSC cell sheets has to be evaluated before clinical application.

## Dentin-Pulp Regeneration

The attempts to induce tissue regeneration in the pulp space have been a long quest. In the early phase, investigators attempted to induce hemorrhage and form blood clots in the canal space of mature teeth in the hope of guiding tissue repair in the canal.[51,52] However, the growth of connective tissue into the canal space was limited and was not real pulp tissue.

Since the isolation and characterization of DPSCs, SHED, and SCAP, dental pulp tissue regeneration has been examined with dental stem cells and various biomate-rials. Cultured DPSCs and SHED are capable of generating a dentin-pulp–like com-plex in vivo when cotransplanted with HA/TCP particles subcutaneously into immunocompromised mice.[21,25] SHED with biodegradable scaffolds seeded onto hu-man tooth slices successfully differentiated into odontoblastlike cells on the dentin surface.[53,54] However, no orthotopic pulplike tissues regenerated in the pulp space with this approach, because of the lack of sufficient blood supply. It has been pro-posed that, because of the concern over vascularization, a stepwise insertion of engi-neered pulp may have to be implemented clinically to achieve the desired pulp tissue regeneration.[55] In addition, many studies suggest that both in vitro and in vivo growth factors can induce regenerative events in the dentin-pulp complex in a similar way to dentin matrix extracts naturally containing these growth factors, including TGF-β and dentin matrix acidic phosphoprotein 1 (DMP1).[56–58] Stem cell–based pulp engineer-ing, cleaning, and shaping of root canals followed by the implantation of vital dental pulp tissue constructs created in the laboratory is suggested for future regenerative endodontic treatment.

## STEM CELL THERAPIES FOR IMMUNE DISEASES

Recent studies highlighted the immunomodulatory properties of MSCs by inhibiting proliferation and function of several major immune cells, including T and B lympho-cytes, DCs, and NK cells, with the association of cytokines. MSC-based therapy is considered to be safe and yields clinical benefit for a variety of immune diseases, such as graft-versus-host disease, SLE, systemic sclerosis (SS), rheumatoid arthritis, Sjögren syndrome, and bisphosphonate-related osteonecrosis of the jaw (BRONJ). The therapeutic mechanisms may involve paracrine secretion of cytokines from MSCs as well as interplay between MSCs and immune cells.

## Systemic Lupus Erythematosus

SLE is a chronic, inflammatory, and febrile systemic disorder of connective tissue with protean manifestations, ranging from minor skin and joint symptoms to severe major organ involvement. It is characterized by the presence of autoreactive T and B lymphocytes, with the generation of pathogenic antibodies directed against a variety of autoantigens, including nuclear and cytoplasmic antigens.

MSC transplant (MSCT) was found to significantly ameliorate lupus nephritis and osteoporosis, and stabilize levels of proinflammatory cytokines in MRL/*lpr* mice, which is an established SLE mode. The mechanisms by which MSCT might ameliorate phenotypes of SLE have been investigated. Most systemically infused MSCs fail to engraft into recipient organs. The success of the MSCT-based therapeutic effects may depend on the cellular and molecular regulation in the recipient after MSCT. MSCT in Fas-deficient MRL/*lpr* mice has been shown to rescue BMMSC function and osteopenia through reducing Th17 levels and the increase of Treg levels.[17] Rebalancing of the autoimmune microenvironment therefore contributes to maintaining long-term therapeutic effects by MSC administration. This experimental evidence also implies that Fas might be able to control cellular components and the release of small extracellular vesicles such as exosomes. Unlike soluble factors such as cytokines and chemokines, recent studies showed that cell-based therapy, a nongenetic approach, is able to rescue impaired MSC function via a protein or microRNA (miRNA) reuse mechanism to restore an epigenetic conversion. Meanwhile, Fas controls miRNA release by exosomes in transplanted MSCs, which regulates DNA methyltransferase expression and causes DNA hypomethylation. Thus, Fas is required to maintain methylation homeostasis in MSCs. Exosomes secreted by donor MSCs contain proteins and miRNAs are reused by recipient cells to restore epigenetic status. MSC administration rescues recipient cell function via cellular component reuse-mediated alteration of intracellular molecular signaling by epigenetic modification, which provides an underlying mechanism on how a single round of MSC infusion yields long-term therapeutic benefits. MSC-based therapy therefore offers a protein/miRNA reuse mechanism that is able to rescue lost gene function in vivo by an epigenetic regulation to achieve therapeutic effects.[59] MSCT in SLE may involve the immunobalance in vivo, such as upregulation of Treg cells associated with a concomitant increase in TGFβ and IL-10, so the balance of Th1 and Th2 is shifted toward Th2, indicated by a higher level of IL-4 and a lower level of IFN-$\gamma$.[60]

Further clinical study in patients with lupus nephritis suggested that allogeneic MSCT is effective in inducing renal remission for both active and refractory lupus nephritis within 12 months, and earlier MSCT may be more efficacious. Primary paracrine factors, such as hepatocyte growth factor (HGF), insulinlike growth factor 1, and vascular endothelial growth factor, may also mediate the process.[61] In terms of the optimum frequency of MSCT, a single MSC transplant at the dose of 1 million MSCs per kilogram of body weight is sufficient to induce disease remission for patients with refractory SLE.[62] Long-term safety and efficacy of MSCT in patients with treatment-resistant SLE were also investigated during a 4-year follow-up, which confirmed the clinical efficacy without any MSCT-related adverse events.[63,64]

### *Systemic Sclerosis*

SS is a chronic multisystem disorder of connective tissue.[65] Both antigen stimulation and genetic susceptibility may contribute to autoimmunity, with consequent early T-cell, B-cell, and fibroblast activation.

In a fibrillin-1 deficiency–induced SS mice model, systemic infusion of MSCs can ameliorate disease phenotypes by inducing transient T-cell apoptosis via the FASL-dependent FAS pathway, triggering macrophages to produce high levels of TGF-β, which in turn upregulates $CD4^+CD25^+Foxp3^+$ Tregs. Eventually, upregulation of Tregs results in immune tolerance and ameliorates disease phenotype.[20,66]

The feasibility, safety, and (most notably) efficacy of allogeneic MSCT in patients with SS have been investigated. Having received an intravenous injection of allogeneic MSCs, a patient with severe refractory SS had a significant decrease in the number of digital ulcers after 3 months.[67] MSCT could induce CD3[+] T-cell apoptosis and Treg upregulation in patients with SS.[68] The first observations were reported in 5 cases. No major side effects or specific abnormalities were observed, including cardiovascular and pulmonary insufficiencies, infection, malignancy, and metabolic disturbances, after follow-ups from 44, 24, 6, 23, and 18 months, respectively, which suggested the safety of MSC therapy in patients with SS.[69]

### Bisphosphonate-related Osteonecrosis of the Jaw

Among the many immune-related diseases in the orofacial region, BRONJ is a critical side effect of bisphosphonate therapy for patients with metastatic cancer or osteoporosis, especially in those who undergo high-dose bisphosphonate and immunosuppressant drug administration. To date, appropriate therapy has not yet been established for the treatment of BRONJ, largely because of a lack of understanding of its pathophysiologic mechanisms. A mouse model of BRONJ-like disease has been developed by the administration of zoledronate and dexamethasone, an immunosuppressant drug, and showed that such BRONJ-like disease in mice is caused by suppression of Tregs and activation of Th17 cells.[70] Note that systemic infusion of MSCs is able to prevent and cure BRONJ-like disease, possibly via induction of peripheral tolerance through inhibition of Th17 cells and increase of Treg levels, thereby supporting the rationale for the use of MSCs as an immunomodulatory approach for BRONJ treatment.[70] In addition, local transplant of MSCs with platelet-rich plasma was reported to alleviate a BRONJ lesion in a patient undergoing alendronate and pamidronate treatment of osteoporosis, with complete healing observed in a 30-month follow-up.[71]

## FUTURE DIRECTION AND CHALLENGES

Human stem cell research has enormous potential for contributing to the understanding and treatment of human biology and disease. Because the biological properties and functions of MSCs are not fully understood, developing an effective approach to prevent or cure human diseases will be difficult. There are several main objectives that need to be addressed before the development of effective MSC-based therapies.

1. Understanding the mechanisms of self-renewal will allow clinicians to regulate adult stem cell growth in vitro to generate sufficient cell numbers for clinical applications. The maintenance or improvement of their stemness is a necessity for the cell expansion process.
2. Understanding the regulation of stem cells during differentiation, specific tissue production, and the specialized extracellular materials required for certain tissues, such as bone, dentin, cartilage, and tendon. The production of the extracellular matrix and its maturation into specialized tissues involve a sequential activation of cascades of signals, which may facilitate the desired tissue regeneration.
3. Understanding the interactions between stem cells and the immune system. Immunosuppressive allogenic MSCs may present an abundant cell source for clinical applications. Further research is needed to determine whether and how allogenic dental MSCs suppress recipient host short-term and long-term immunorejection.

In the future, a more widespread, cost-effective, and regular use of MSCs for cell-based therapy must be sustained by an efficient, reliable, and reproducible MSC expansion system. Moreover, in order to be good manufacturing practices (GMP)-compliant, the ex vivo expansion of MSCs will require clinical-grade systems, as well as effective standards and methodologies for preclinical safety and efficacy evaluation, product characterization, and guidelines for cell-based therapeutic applications.[72]

## REFERENCES

1. Takahashi K, Yamanaka S. Induction of pluripotent stem cells from mouse embryonic and adult fibroblast cultures by defined factors. Cell 2006;126(4):663–76.

2. Friedenstein AJ, Petrakova KV, Kurolesova AI, et al. Heterotopic of bone marrow. Analysis of precursor cells for osteogenic and hematopoietic tissues. Transplantation 1968;6(2):230–47.

3. Liu Y, Wang S, Shi S. The role of recipient T cells in mesenchymal stem cell-based tissue regeneration. Int J Biochem Cell Biol 2012;44(11):2044–50.

4. Driskell RR, Clavel C, Rendl M, et al. Hair follicle dermal papilla cells at a glance. J Cell Sci 2011;124(Pt 8):1179–82.

5. Chai Y, Maxson RE. Recent advances in craniofacial morphogenesis. Dev Dyn 2006;235:2353–75.

6. Chai Y, Jiang X, Ito Y, et al. Fate of the mammalian cranial neural crest during tooth and mandibular morphogenesis. Development 2000;127:1671–9.

7. Huang GT, Gronthos S, Shi S. Mesenchymal stem cells derived from dental tissues vs. those from other sources: their biology and role in regenerative medicine. J Dent Res 2009;88(9):792–806.

8. Yamaza T, Kentaro A, Chen C, et al. Immunomodulatory properties of stem cells from human exfoliated deciduous teeth. Stem Cell Res Ther 2010;1(1):5.

9. Dominici M, Le Blanc K, Mueller I, et al. Minimal criteria for defining multipotent mesenchymal stromal cells. The International Society for Cellular Therapy position statement. Cytotherapy 2006;8(4):315–7.

10. Konttinen YT, Kaivosoja E, Stegaev V, et al. Chapter 2: extracellular matrix and tissue regeneration. Regenerative medicine: from protocol to patient. Springer Dordrecht Heidelberg London New York; 2013. p. 21–78.

11. Shi S, Gronthos S, Chen S, et al. Bone formation by human postnatal bone marrow stromal stem cells is enhanced by telomerase expression. Nat Biotechnol 2002;20:587–91.

12. Gronthos S, Chen S, Wang CY, et al. Telomerase accelerates osteogenesis of bone marrow stromal stem cells by regulation of CBFA1, osterix, and osteocalcin. J Bone Miner Res 2003;18:716–22.

13. Pittenger MF, Mackay AM, Beck SC, et al. Multilineage potential of adult human mesenchymal stem cells. Science 1999;284(5411):143–7.

14. Nauta AJ, Fibbe WE. Immunomodulatory properties of mesenchymal stromal cells. Blood 2007;110(10):3499–506.

15. Di Nicola M, Carlo-Stella C, Magni M, et al. Human bone marrow stromal cells suppress T-lymphocyte proliferation induced by cellular or nonspecific mitogenic stimuli. Blood 2002;99(10):3838–43.

16. Aggarwal S, Pittenger MF. Human mesenchymal stem cells modulate allogeneic immune cell responses. Blood 2005;105(4):1815–22.

17. Sun L, Akiyama K, Zhang H, et al. Mesenchymal stem cell transplantation reverses multiorgan dysfunction in systemic lupus erythematosus mice and humans. Stem Cells 2009;27(6):1421–32.

18. Fontenot JD, Gavin MA, Rudensky AY. Foxp3 programs the development and function of CD4+CD25+ regulatory T cells. Nat Immunol 2003;4(4):330–6.
19. Di Ianni M, Del Papa B, De Ioanni M, et al. Mesenchymal cells recruit and regulate T regulatory cells. Exp Hematol 2008;36(3):309–18.
20. Akiyama K, Chen C, Wang D, et al. Mesenchymal stem cell induced immunoregulation involves FAS ligand/FAS-mediated T cell apoptosis. Cell Stem Cell 2012; 10(5):544–55.
21. Gronthos S, Mankani M, Brahim J, et al. Postnatal human dental pulp stem cells (DPSCs) in vitro and in vivo. Proc Natl Acad Sci U S A 2000;97(25):13625–30.
22. Huang G, Sonoyama W, Chen J, et al. In vitro characterization of human dental pulp cells: various isolation methods and culturing environments. Cell Tissue Res 2006;324(2):225–36.
23. Huang GT, Shagramanova K, Chan SW. Formation of odontoblast like cells from cultured human dental pulp cells on dentin in vitro. J Endod 2006;32(11): 1066–73.
24. Batouli S, Miura M, Brahim J, et al. Comparison of stem cell mediated osteogenesis and dentinogenesis. J Dent Res 2003;82(12):976–81.
25. Miura M, Gronthos S, Zhao M, et al. SHED: stem cells from human exfoliated deciduous teeth. Proc Natl Acad Sci U S A 2003;100(10):5807–12.
26. Kerkis I, Kerkis A, Dozortsev D, et al. Isolation and characterization of a population of immature dental pulp stem cells expressing OCT-4 and other embryonic stem cell markers. Cells Tissues Organs 2006;184(3–4):105–16.
27. Seo BM, Miura M, Gronthos S, et al. Investigation of multipotent postnatal stem cells from human periodontal ligament. Lancet 2004;364(9429):149–55.
28. Sonoyama W, Liu Y, Yamaza T, et al. Characterization of the apical papilla and its residing stem cells from human immature permanent teeth: a pilot study. J Endod 2008;34(2):166–71.
29. Morsczeck C, Götz W, Schierholz J, et al. Isolation of precursor cells (PCs) from human dental follicle of wisdom teeth. Matrix Biol 2005;24(2):155–65.
30. Zhang Q, Shi S, Liu Y, et al. Mesenchymal stem cells derived from human gingiva are capable of immunomodulatory functions and ameliorate inflammation related tissue destruction in experimental colitis. J Immunol 2009;183(12):7787–98.
31. Yamaza T, Ren G, Akiyama K, et al. Mouse mandible contains distinctive mesenchymal stem cells. J Dent Res 2011;90(3):317–24.
32. Zhang W, Walboomers XF, Shi S, et al. Multilineage differentiation potential of stem cells derived from human dental pulp after cryopreservation. Tissue Eng 2006;12(10):2813–23.
33. Pierdomenico L, Bonsi L, Calvitti M, et al. Multipotent mesenchymal stem cells with immunosuppressive activity can be easily isolated from dental pulp. Transplantation 2005;80(6):836–42.
34. Liu Y, Chen C, Liu S, et al. Acetylsalicylic acid treatment improves differentiation and immunomodulation of SHED. J Dent Res 2015;94(1):209–18.
35. Liu Y, Wang L, Liu S, et al. Transplantation of SHED presents bone loss in the early phase of ovariectomy-induced osteoporosis. J Dent Res 2014;93(11):1124–32.
36. Xu X, Chen C, Akiyama K, et al. Gingivae contain neural-crest- and mesoderm-derived mesenchymal stem cells. J Dent Res 2013;92(9):825–32.
37. Ding G, Wang W, Liu Y, et al. Effect of cryopreservation on biological and immunological properties of stem cells from apical papilla. J Cell Physiol 2010;223(2): 415–22.
38. Wada N, Menicanin D, Shi S, et al. Immunomodulatory properties of human periodontal ligament stem cells. J Cell Physiol 2009;219(3):667–76.

39. Chamberlain G, Fox J, Ashton B, et al. Concise review: mesenchymal stem cells: their phenotype, differentiation capacity, immunological features, and potential for homing. Stem Cells 2007;25(11):2739–49.

40. Bi Y, Ehirchiou D, Kilts TM, et al. Identification of tendon stem/progenitor cells and the role of the extracellular matrix in their niche. Nat Med 2007;13(10):1219–27.

41. Brivanlou AH, Gage FH, Jaenisch R, et al. Stem cells. Setting standards for human embryonic stem cells. Science 2003;300:913–6.

42. Honda MJ, Ohara T, Sumita Y, et al. Preliminary study of tissue-engineered odontogenesis in the canine jaw. J Oral Maxillofac Surg 2006;64(2):283–9.

43. Kuo TF, Huang AT, Chang HH, et al. Regeneration of dentin-pulp complex with cementum and periodontal ligament formation using dental bud cells in gelatin-chondroitin-hyaluronan tri-copolymer scaffold in swine. J Biomed Mater Res A 2007;86(4):1062–8.

44. Sonoyama W, Liu Y, Fang D, et al. Mesenchymal stem cell-mediated functional tooth regeneration in swine. PLoS One 2006;1(1):e79.

45. Wei F, Song T, Ding G, et al. Functional tooth restoration by allogeneic mesenchymal stem cell-based bio-root regeneration in swine. Stem Cells Dev 2013; 22(12):1752–62.

46. Ding G, Liu Y, Wang W, et al. Allogeneic periodontal ligament stem cell therapy for periodontitis in swine. Stem Cells 2010;28(10):1829–38.

47. Chen FM, Gao LN, Tian BM, et al. Treatment of periodontal intrabony defects using autologous periodontal ligament stem cells: a randomized clinical trial. Stem Cell Res Ther 2016;7(1):33.

48. Flores MG, Hasegawa M, Yamato M, et al. Cementum-periodontal ligament complex regeneration using the cell sheet technique. J Periodont Res 2008;43(3): 364–71.

49. Yang Z, Jin F, Zhang X, et al. Tissue engineering of cementum/periodontal-ligament complex using a novel three-dimensional pellet cultivation system for human periodontal ligament stem cells. Tissue Eng Part C Methods 2009;15(4): 571–81.

50. Feng F, Akiyama K, Liu Y, et al. Utility of PDL progenitors for in vivo tissue regeneration: a report of 3 cases. Oral Dis 2010;16(1):20–8.

51. Ostby BN. The role of the blood clot in endodontic therapy. An experimental histologic study. Acta Odontol Scand 1961;19:324–53.

52. Myers WC, Fountain SB. Dental pulp regeneration aided by blood and blood substitutes after experimentally induced periapical infection. Oral Surg Oral Med Oral Pathol 1974;37(3):441–50.

53. Cordeiro MM, Dong Z, Kaneko T, et al. Dental pulp tissue engineering with stem cells from exfoliated deciduous teeth. J Endod 2008;34(8):962–9.

54. Sakai VT, Zhang Z, Dong Z, et al. SHED differentiate into functional odontoblasts and endothelium. J Dent Res 2010;89(8):791–6.

55. Huang GT, Sonoyama W, Liu Y, et al. The hidden treasure in apical papilla: the potential role in pulp/dentin regeneration and bio-root engineering. J Endod 2008;34(6):645–51.

56. Sloan AJ, Perry H, Matthews JB, et al. Transforming growth factor-beta isoform expression in mature human molar teeth and carious molar teeth. Histochem J 2000;32(4):247–52.

57. Smith AJ, Matthews JB, Hall RC. Transforming growth factor-beta1 (TGF-beta1) in dentine matrix. Ligand activation and receptor expression. Eur J Oral Sci 1998; 106:179–84.

58. Prescott RS, Alsanea R, Fayad MI, et al. In vivo generation of dental pulp-like tissue by using dental pulp stem cells, a collagen scaffold, and dentin matrix protein 1 after subcutaneous transplantation in mice. J Endod 2008;34(4):421–6.

59. Liu S, Liu D, Chen C, et al. MSC transplantation improves osteopenia via epigenetic regulation of notch signaling in lupus. Cell Metab 2015;22(4):606–18.

60. Sun L, Wang D, Liang J, et al. Umbilical cord mesenchymal stem cell transplantation in severe and refractory systemic lupus erythematosus. Arthritis Rheum 2010;62(8):2467–75.

61. Gu F, Wang D, Zhang H, et al. Allogeneic mesenchymal stem cell transplantation for lupus nephritis patients refractory to conventional therapy. Clin Rheumatol 2014;33(11):1611–9.

62. Wang D, Akiyama K, Zhang H, et al. Double allogenic mesenchymal stem cells transplantations could not enhance therapeutic effect compared with single transplantation in systemic lupus erythematosus. Clin Dev Immunol 2012;2012: 273291.

63. Liang J, Zhang H, Hua B, et al. Allogenic mesenchymal stem cells transplantation in refractory systemic lupus erythematosus: a pilot clinical study. Ann Rheum Dis 2010;69(8):1423–9.

64. Wang D, Zhang H, Liang J, et al. Allogeneic mesenchymal stem cell transplantation in severe and refractory systemic lupus erythematosus: 4 years of experience. Cell Transplant 2013;22(12):2267–77.

65. Chen C, Akiyama K, Wang D, et al. mTOR inhibition rescues osteopenia in mice with systemic sclerosis. J Exp Med 2015;212(1):73–91.

66. Chen C, Akiyama K, Yamaza T, et al. Telomerase governs immunomodulatory properties of mesenchymal stem cells by regulating FAS ligand expression. EMBO Mol Med 2014;6(3):322–34.

67. van Laar JM, Farge D, Sont JK, et al. Autologous hematopoietic stem cell transplantation vs intravenous pulse cyclophosphamide in diffuse cutaneous systemic sclerosis: a randomized clinical trial. JAMA 2014;311(24):2490–8.

68. Christopeit M, Schendel M, Föll J, et al. Marked improvement of severe progressive systemic sclerosis after transplantation of mesenchymal stem cells from an allogeneic haploidentical-related donor mediated by ligation of CD137L. Leukemia 2008;22(5):1062–4.

69. Keyszer G, Christopeit M, Fick S, et al. Treatment of severe progressive systemic sclerosis with transplantation of mesenchymal stromal cells from allogeneic related donors: report of five cases. Arthritis Rheum 2011;63(8):2540–2.

70. Kikuiri T, Kim I, Yamaza T, et al. Cell based immunotherapy with mesenchymal stem cells cures bisphosphonate-related osteonecrosis of the jaw-like disease in mice. J Bone Miner Res 2010;25(7):1668–79.

71. Cella L, Oppici A, Arbasi M, et al. Autologous bone marrow stem cell intralesional transplantation repairing bisphosphonate related osteonecrosis of the jaw. Head Face Med 2011;7:16.

72. Kirouac DC, Zandstra PW. The systematic production of cells for cell therapies. Cell Stem Cell 2008;3(4):369–81.

# Index

Note: Page numbers of article titles are in **boldface** type.

Dent Clin N Am 61 (2017) 173–177
http://dx.doi.org/10.1016/S0011-8532(16)30114-8
0011-8532/17

**dental.theclinics.com**

# Moving?

## Make sure your subscription moves with you!

To notify us of your new address, find your **Clinics Account Number** (located on your mailing label above your name), and contact customer service at:

**Email: journalscustomerservice-usa@elsevier.com**

**800-654-2452** (subscribers in the U.S. & Canada)
**314-447-8871** (subscribers outside of the U.S. & Canada)

**Fax number: 314-447-8029**

**Elsevier Health Sciences Division**
**Subscription Customer Service**
**3251 Riverport Lane**
**Maryland Heights, MO 63043**

*To ensure uninterrupted delivery of your subscription, please notify us at least 4 weeks in advance of move.

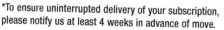
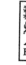

Printed and bound by CPI Group (UK) Ltd, Croydon, CR0 4YY

07/10/2024

01040500-0016